ER Nurse:
The Warrior Within

Bruised, But Still Standing

Jocelyn Cerrudo Sese

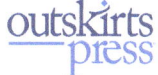

ER Nurse: The Warrior Within
Bruised, But Still Standing
All Rights Reserved.
Copyright © 2021 Jocelyn Cerrudo Sese
v4.0

The opinions expressed in this manuscript are solely the opinions of the author and do not represent the opinions or thoughts of the publisher. The author has represented and warranted full ownership and/or legal right to publish all the materials in this book.

This book may not be reproduced, transmitted, or stored in whole or in part by any means, including graphic, electronic, or mechanical without the express written consent of the publisher except in the case of brief quotations embodied in critical articles and reviews.

Outskirts Press, Inc.
http://www.outskirtspress.com

Paperback ISBN: 978-1-9772-4324-9
Hardback ISBN: 978-1-9772-4387-4

Cover Photo © 2021 www.gettyimages.com. All rights reserved - used with permission.

Outskirts Press and the "OP" logo are trademarks belonging to Outskirts Press, Inc.

PRINTED IN THE UNITED STATES OF AMERICA

DEDICATION

To my family,
All that I am
All that I will be
All, because of you.

To all nurses,
At the end of the day,
You all made a difference.
That's your legacy.

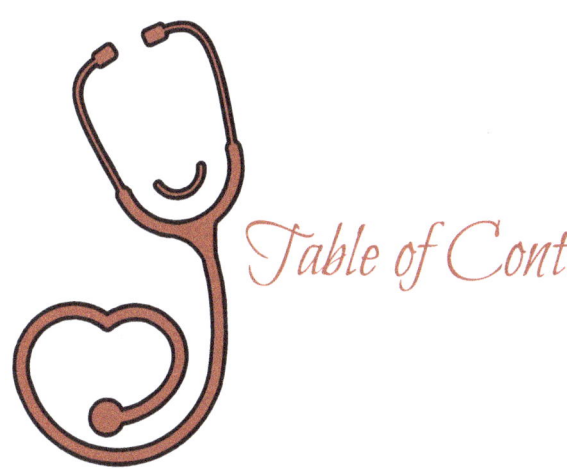

Table of Contents

Part 1: ER Vignettes

Happiness... to an ER Nurse 3

When Nurses Cry 5

Finding my Joy in Nursing: Knowing my Whys 8

Nurse, Can You Tell My Story? 13

Organized Chaos 20

When One of Our Own Is the Patient: Anna's Story 22

"You must be kidding!!!!" 26

Papi: A Migrant Story 30

"Oh, No! Trauma Again?" 33

The Heart Remembers 38

ED Odd 41

Ignorance and Bigotry 45

Only in the ER 48

The Holiday Heart 52

The Baby is Coming 54

"No More Abuse!" 56

My Human 58

Nursing, Thirty-Eight Years Ago… 61

Life in the ER 66

Leigh's syndrome: A Day in the Pediatric ED 71

Making a Difference as an ED Nurse 75

Part 2: ED Covid-19 Nursing Diaries

ED Nurse Covid Diaries 83

Pandemic Reflection: One Year Later 111

Part 3: In the Future

Nurse of the Future, 2025 115

ED nursing: In the Year 2030 121

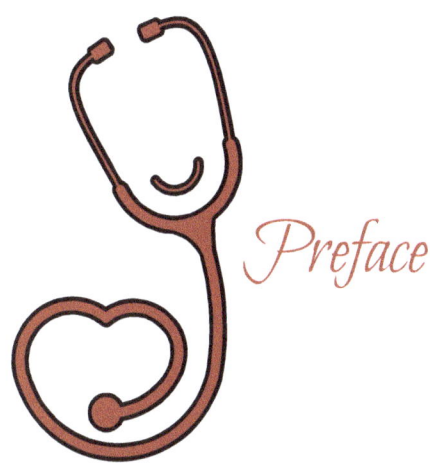

Preface

I am an ER nurse and I have many stories to share after thirty-one years of ER nursing. The ER is both my war zone and my sanctuary. My truths and lived experience are just a glimpse into the world of trauma, crises, diseases, and human sufferings.

The stories at the frontlines are outrageous, funny and sad, tragic and inspirational. Over the years, I survived the psychological land mines by purposefully celebrating the emotional rewards and joys of being an ER nurse. I fought a good fight. I kept my sanity and overcame my vulnerabilities to emerge triumphant. I am battle-scarred but stronger, bruised but still standing.

The year 2020 was a year like no other. The Covid-19 pandemic challenged our resources and affected us in so many ways both known and unknown. Although the sad memories continue to haunt us to this very day, there are so many stories of triumph and resilience in healthcare. I am never prouder to be a nurse.

With these stories, I want to magnify the nurses' voice, to define and exemplify the resilience of the frontliners. I believe that there is always something in my stories that will resonate with any nurse or any caregiver. I hope to inspire future nurses and to reassure current nurses that they make a difference in somebody's lives.

This book is a labor of love. It is an expression of my gratitude to the nursing profession. My experiences have forever changed me. I am a better person. I hope you understand my "Why".

All the stories in Parts 1 and 2 are true, except in the "My Human" story. The names and identifiers were changed to protect patient privacy and confidentiality.

The stories in Part 3 are creative figments of my imagination. Because they're set in the future, I am curious to revisit these stories when the time comes.

Jocelyn Cerrudo Sese,
RN, MSN, CEN, TCRN, NE-BC, NHDP-BC

"I don't know how any nurse does what they do, but aside from that, what really struck me was that in the middle of all these horrible, tragic moments, you would see a nurse lean over and just say, "hey, I've got you", or give somebody water, and not just give it to them, but do it in a way that showed they cared for them. - Award-winning filmmaker Carolyn Jones

Part 1:
ER Vignettes

I told myself in 1990 that I will stay in ER Nursing for two years only.

I never left.

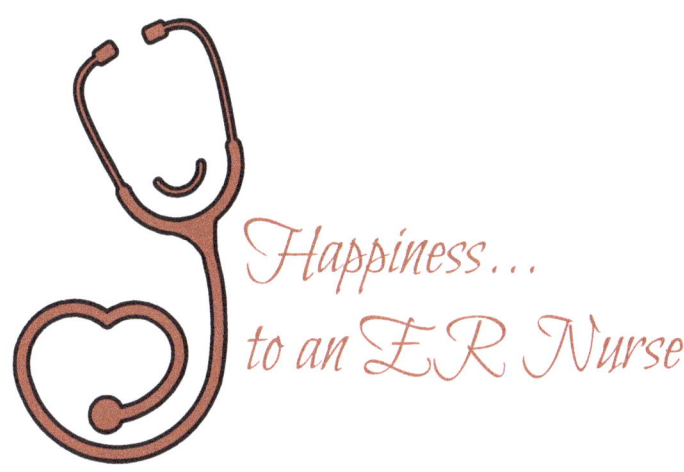

Happiness... to an ER Nurse

An ER nurse is of a special breed. Our sense of humor is off-beat and off-centric to most, especially to those not in the nursing profession. But even among other nurses, we have acquired an unfair reputation; we are branded as aggressive and rude, and most in-patient nurses regard us as too cold and not as caring.

Hey missy, if you have to deal with the never-ending traffic of patients and the constant stressors, you probably would have run far, far away like Speedy Gonzalez. Just try to spend an hour in our shoes and see if you can handle the stress.

Maybe we are crazy, maybe we are just adrenaline-junkies, but we have learned to appreciate the little things that make life in the ER not just tolerable but have actually induced a chuckle or two. To survive, we found delight in the simple pleasures of ER life.

Tongue-in-cheek humor; anything to brighten the day and to lighten the load.

Happiness... to an ER nurse:

1. Being relieved on time because your relief found parking on time.
2. Having the right team with you, although you were short-staffed.
3. Receiving a thank you from that difficult patient who almost made you forget you're a nurse.
4. Saving a life because you dared to question a wrong order.
5. Seeing the hallway filled with stretchers; that means the ED is empty.
6. Getting patients with great veins.
7. Finishing the shift without being cursed, hit at or hit on.
8. Getting a typed list of medications at triage instead of two bagful of medications that needed to be sorted out.
9. Changing the child's pain scale from 10 to 0, and finally getting a reprieve from the demanding parents.
10. Connecting the dots on a puzzling case in the ED and coming up with the presumptive diagnosis before the doctor did.
11. Witnessing the facial droop disappear after the thrombolytic did its magic.
12. Catching a baby before it hits the floor (a lucky catch since the mother initially denied she's pregnant.)

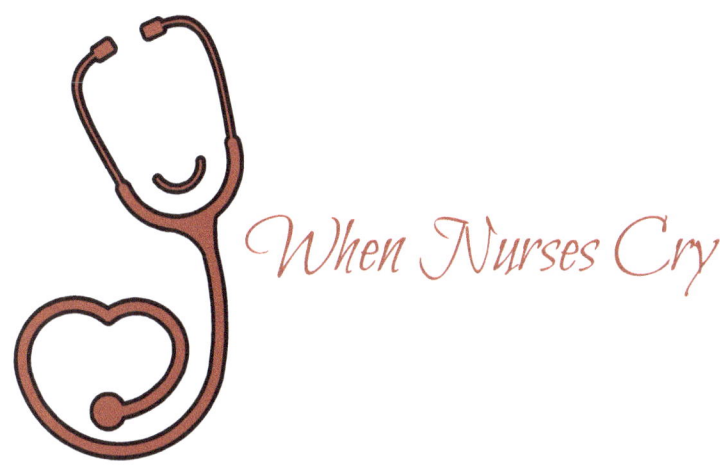

When Nurses Cry

The viral picture of a doctor grieving after a patient died resonated with me. The loss was palpable; the helplessness was disturbing. It has struck a chord in every other person who works in the medical field. A poignant image that happens all the time, it is replicated in the privacy of the staff lounges, in the restrooms, in the offices, anywhere nurses and doctors are able to escape for a few moments to grieve.

I have cried many times in my nursing career. For those we have lost and those we cannot help.

I spent my first four years in the US as a nurse in a chronic care hospital in Roosevelt Island in New York. My first patient death experience was an end-stage renal disease patient who suffered a cardiac arrest. The other nurses who helped me do the post-mortem care were as distraught as me. Our tears blended with the bath water as we washed the patient's uremic skin and combed her gray matted hair.

There were more patients in that unit who died after her. The patients were our family… and every time one passed away, we cried with the rest of the staff. Most of the time, the nurses were the only ones who mourned their passing because the families had long abandoned the patients.

When I started to work in the emergency department, I taught myself to be stoic. It was my shield against the pain of tragic loss, my armor to protect my heart from shredding whenever a patient died. I could not afford to be burned-out. The compassion and empathy remained, but breaking down in tears is something I avoided.

Death is a constant in the emergency room. Some of those deaths were hard and brutal, unexpected and difficult to accept. However, there were some deaths that were almost a welcome event, especially for those chronically-ill patients who lived through extreme pain. For them, death released them from hell on earth.

Every so often, something pierced through the thick armor I built around my emotions.

I cried for one young man who came in traumatic arrest after a motorcycle crash.

I cried with a wife and her son when the patient died after they signed the Do Not Resuscitate papers. The son just reconciled with his estranged father.

I cried when the cardiac ultrasound revealed no cardiac activity. The patient was one of our own nurses who came in cardiac arrest after collapsing on her way in to work.

I cried with the elderly husband who grieved for his wife of fifty years.

I cried when a six-month old baby drowned in bath water.

I cried with the nursing staff when one of our favorite "regular' drunks died from hypothermia.

I cried when the seventy-year-old woman who swallowed cocaine bags to earn money for her daughter's cancer treatment died on the way to the OR.

I cried when a young pregnant mother succumbed to her injuries after she was struck down by a forklift. I cried for her baby who survived but had brain damage.

I cried when a bullied teen-ager jumped to his death.

After I cried, I went back to work. Such is the life of those who work in the medical field. There is always someone who needs our help, someone who needs the narcotic Dilaudid. Breathe in, breathe out. There was not enough time to lament the loss of life because there are so many more who need our attention.

I Cried

**I have cried many times in my nursing career.
For those we have lost and those we cannot help.
After I cried, I went back to work.
Such is the life of those who work in the
medical field.
There is always someone who needs our help,
someone who needs the Dilaudid.**

Jocelyn Cerrudo Sese

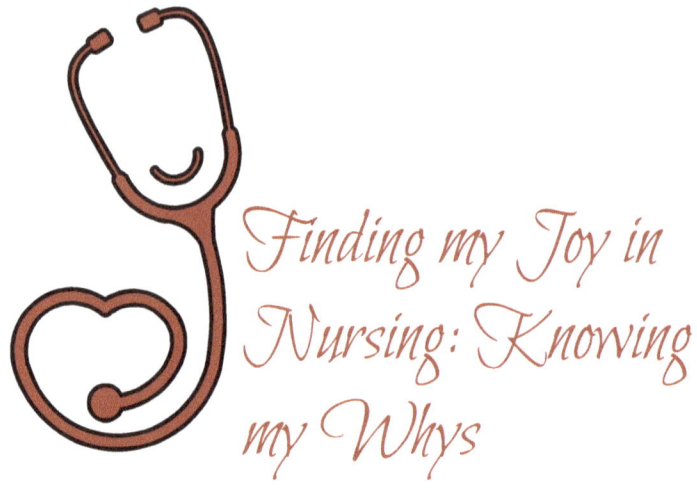

Finding my Joy in Nursing: Knowing my Whys

Life's ebb and flow can sometimes numb you in just going through the motion without the conscious enjoyment of living. The stress of work and personal lives can often leech out happiness in one or both worlds.

"Plan your joy", Michelle Obama said. We need to care for ourselves and to take the time to invigorate and refresh ourselves. There needs to be a good work-life balance in order to survive physically, mentally, and emotionally. Self-care is being mindful of our needs so we can in turn care for others.

I actively and deliberately plan my joy outside work. Whether planning the itinerary for a vacation or just enjoying a no-stress-and-waking-up-late-week-end, I seek those things that give me comfort and happiness. Good books, funny movies, soothing music, food trips around Queens with my son and family, and indulging in my joy of writing. My guilty pleasures are to explore the things that are meaningful and give me joy. Even just having a quiet time lounging in my sofa with the mood music on and the dog snoring at my feet. There is a thoughtful consideration to enjoy my days off work in order to recharge myself.

Because I spend a lot of my wake time at work, I also plan my joy when I'm working in the hospital. Unfortunately, I have seen some co-workers who allowed their work to drain the joy in their lives and they end up burned-out and bitter, sometimes because they felt trapped in a job that no longer sustains them and sometimes because they are afraid to spread their wings and find an environment that gives them joy. I am lucky than most because I truly have enjoyed my nursing journey.

The emergency department itself can be chaotic and stressful. This is the nature of my work; there are sad times when some of our patients die but there is joy when we are able to give someone a second chance at life. In all my years of nursing, from my first job as a staff nurse at a chronic care hospital to my current role as director of nursing in a busy emergency department in Manhattan, I made and still make a conscious effort to enjoy these moments of joy. Being joyful is not being artificial and unrealistically pollyannaish. I would rather think of it as being Optimistic, not just a Value of the Month. It is just knowing that we can reframe our minds to find meaning and purpose and joy however stressful the work environment is.

As a nursing leader, I feel the responsibility to help my nurses re-discover the joy in their work. There are financial constraints in staffing, but there is always something to do to empower our nurses to enjoy their work, even if sometimes the trials to both body and spirit can be challenging. I would like my staff to feel that they belong and they are appreciated and that they matter. One day, a nurse stopped me to complain about the admission boarders in the ED, those patients take out their frustrations on the nurses because they were waiting for inpatient beds. I gently asked her if she is asking to transfer to another unit. As I actually expected, she burst out laughing and said, *"Hahaha, I am just venting. I love my patients and I love my co-workers. I know you are doing your best to staff the unit and I love you as my leader. Thanks for listening."*.

I celebrate the work of every healthcare person in the hospital. A single person can make a difference. At our leadership retreat, the testimony of a trauma survivor touched my heart. She was a pedestrian struck patient who sustained multiple fractures and injuries. She recounted very candidly her ordeal back to recovery and gave thoughtful and honest suggestions on how we can make things better for the next patient. She was thankful for the many healthcare workers who made a difference in her care. She spoke about simple acts of kindness like the ice cream from a dietary aide and the shampoo that the trauma coordinator helped her with. She remembered the good, the bad, and the ugly, but she earnestly spoke of the things that lifted her heart.

As all other nurses, I live for the unexpected Thank You. One elderly man thanked me for staying with his anxious wife while he parked the car. It was just a simple gesture, just a few minutes of my time. To this couple, this meant that the wife's anxiety did not unravel to a full-blown panic attack. The elderly man didn't know that just a few minutes ago, I came from assisting in a cardiac arrest of a young man who succumbed from an overdose. The "thank yous" are our emotional rewards, Two simple words that gave me joy that day.

Many years ago, a boy was hit in the middle of his chest with a baseball. He went into cardiac arrest, in commotio cordis, and was rushed to the OR. Three weeks later, the boy returned to the ED with his mom to thank the ED and surgical staff for the heroic efforts of saving him. The boy named Pedro beamed as he was surrounded by weeping nurses.

There are many moments of happiness in the midst of the darkness in the medical world. We have saved many patients, eased the sufferings of those we cannot save, and touched many lives along the way. Caring for someone does have many rewards.

The comedian Michael Jr. explained, "When you know your 'why' then your 'what' has more impact, because you're working towards your purpose." In his video, he showed a man who discovered his WHY and sang Amazing Grace with his heart.

The author Simon Sinek wrote that that "it is only when you understand your "why" (or your purpose) that you'll be more capable of pursuing the things that give you fulfillment". A purpose-driven life clears your pathway and provides direction to your life. This happens when you find your joy in your life.

My joy is in the numerous little ways that validate me as a nurse. The ways we make a difference strengthen me amidst the sadness and chaos; a reminder why I am a nurse. The reason WHY I stay and keep on going is because it is indeed a blessing to be part of a service profession that gives patients more than just a second chance.

Moments like these give us the joys in our work. Nurses

appreciate the simple pleasures- a thank you from a patient or a colleague, a life saved, recognition for a job well done, and a chuckle shared with co-workers. I do not have to reflect long and hard to remember the joys in my nursing life. **This is my "WHY", my 'IKIGAI' or "my reason for being".**

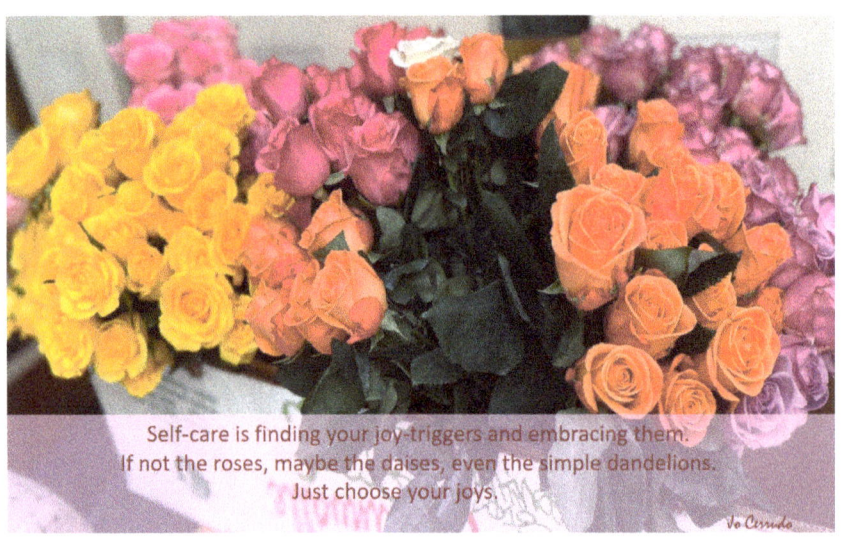

Self-care is finding your joy-triggers and embracing them. If not the roses, maybe the daises, even the simple dandelions. Just choose your joys.

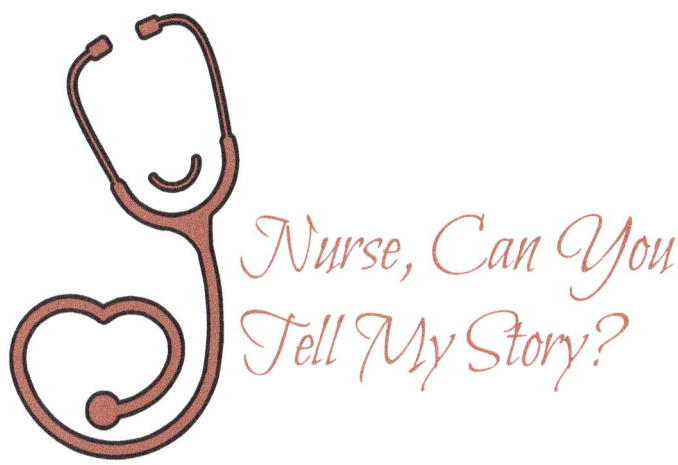

Nurse, Can You Tell My Story?

Email thread

11/26/15

Hi Ms. Cerrudo,

On this Thanksgiving, I write to simply say "thank you". I randomly come across your blog. I'm not in the medical field, but know it well - as a patient. A few years ago, I was taken into surgery for an emergent surgery. The doctors discovered several masses. Unfortunately, the hepatic artery was nicked during the case and I began bleeding profusely- I subsequently coded twice during the case and it was a very skilled RN that helped perform open cardiac massage. After several weeks of intense recovery, I made it home.

I now face a second major surgery in a month to attempt to repair a thoracoabdominal aortic aneurysm that is pressuring both the spinal cord and diaphragm. Additionally, they will attempt to remove some metastatic lesions on the upper and lower GI tract. They have estimated a 16-hour case with a 70% intra-op mortality rate.

I write to you to thank you for sharing all of your stories to exemplify how important nurses are in the direst of situations. I was able to obtain authorization for an observer during my upcoming surgery and was wondering if you might want to observe - I think so much good could come out of you sharing my story and to re-emphasize that medicine is a balance of technical skill, compassion and humanity. I could think of nobody better to tell that story.

I want to specifically thank the nurses. They are my comforters: the ER nurses, the ICU nurses, and the OR nurses. I thanked the doctors enough, but the nurses don't get enough credit.

11/27/15

Hi Mike,

My heart goes out to you. Despite all that you have gone through, you still managed to recognize the contribution of nurses to your care. I have never received a request from a patient for me to share their story. It will be an honor and a privilege for me to assist you in any way I can.

Let me know how I can help. When is your surgery? I will be leaving for a 3-week vacation in January. I wish I can see you before then. I would really like to meet you.

11/29/15

Hi Jocelyn,

Thank you for getting back to me. Would you be open talking to me very soon? I would love to tell you of the many ways that the nurses made a difference in my care. How they comforted me when I was anxious; when I just needed someone to talk to. A nurse stayed with me until I fell asleep. Can I send you my case study?

12/6/15

Hi Mike,

I read your case study. Words fail me because I cannot imagine how difficult it is for you and your family. If you would like to discuss this with me, I would be available this Saturday before the holiday rush. In mid-January, I will be out of the country on vacation. I do want to speak to you by phone or in person, if you're up to it. Your story needs to be told.

(In truth, I was so touched by Mike's trust in sharing his case study. He's not even thirty yet, and he has gone through a lot. The doctors removed some lesions on his gastrointestinal tract. The names of the OR staff were redacted in the operative report. The case details chronicled the whole session. The assisting surgeon prayed for spiritual guidance for the OR staff. She also prayed for the patient- for his comfort and peace of mind so that he will feel the "hedge of angels surrounding" him. She also prayed that the lessons from this case study will benefit others in the future.

Except for a month's stint in the operating room as a nursing student, I have not known much about how much stressful it is to work in the OR setting; how tenuous a life is; how in one instant, patient can bleed out from a ruptured artery. The attending surgeon stepped out twice to inform Mike's parents of complications during surgery. Each single time, the attending came back with the family's decision for a full code. The OR surgeons, physician assistants, nurses, and scrub techs all rooted for Mike, and he survived. No neurological complication from the two episodes of cardiac arrest- one from ventricular fibrillation and one from an asystolic rhythm.)

12/10/15

Hi Jocelyn, Was there anything in-particular that resonated with you about my case? Have you ever had to perform compressions on the table during a non-emergent case? Both external and internal?

12/11/15

Dear Mike,

Several things that resonated with me about your case:

1. *Your resilience. Your strength comes through loud and clear. The operative report was so graphic and so detailed, especially in the resuscitation efforts. Everything was so surreal.*

2. Your spirituality. I did not even know that prayers are held right there in the OR.

I have been an ER nurse for about 25 years. I spent the last 12 years as an educator. I have done my fair share of external cardiac compressions. When I was still doing trauma, I had assisted in cardiac resuscitation using the internal defibrillation paddles, but I have not done an internal cardiac massage. The closest I have ever come to seeing this was when the trauma surgeons opened up an eight-year-old boy who was hit by a baseball in his chest. To this day, I still get goosebumps when I remember the day the boy came back to the ED several weeks later, alive and well. I have never been so happy seeing the healed scar on his chest.

(In fact, I wanted to tell Mike how grateful I am that we were able to talk over the phone. I felt emotional hearing his voice, especially since I realize that his impending surgery is complicated. He expressed optimism, but I sensed that he was resigned to the fact that he might not make it this time. With the 70% intra-op mortality rate, the odds are against him. We made another appointment to talk again. We did not have a chance to speak again since he was busy with more tests).

1/12/16

Mike, In a few days' time, you will undergo surgery again. I am sorry that I would not be able to be there for you because I am boarding the plane to see my family. I will pray for you. Would you email me back when you have recovered? Be strong.

1/20/16

Mike, I pray that the operation was a success. Please email me back.

(I called him from overseas a day after his surgery and several days later. The phone just rang and rang. I prayed that he was just busy recovering).

2/26/16

Hi Mike,

This is Jocelyn. It has been a while since we corresponded. I am not sure what happened since then. Can you please e-mail me back?

3/8/16

Mike, are you there? I tried to call your phone, but it was not in service. I also tried to google your name for any news but did not get anything.

11/26/16

Mike, it has been a year since you e-mailed me. I am afraid that it is not good news since I haven't heard from you. I do not want to intrude on your family's privacy so although I know your real name, I couldn't reach out to your family. Are they even aware that you want your story shared with the world? I *do not know you personally, but I am convinced that for whatever little time you have on earth (I feared the worst), you have enriched the lives of those around you.*

I am humbled that you chose me to tell your story. You wanted to honor the nurses. Instead, I honor you.

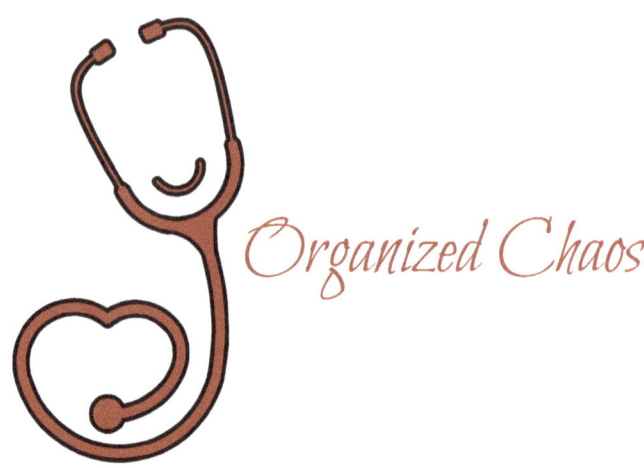

Organized Chaos

At Triage...

EMS#1: "My patient inhaled cockroach spray. You have to triage me first."

EMS#2: "I was here first. My patient was found sleeping in the subway station and the police couldn't wake him up."

Patient: "Nurse, you can't keep me against my will. I know my rights. I'll call my lawyers."

Clerk: "Triage nurse, you have a call from the clinic on line three."

Tech: "Did you order these bloods? I need your signature."

Family: "Miss, did you see my father? He's the one with the rash."

Police: "When will the doctor see this perp? She's got to sew him up before I can take him back to Central Booking."

Visitor: "How do I get to the clinic?"

Clerk: "The head nurse is in a meeting. Can you answer this call?"

EMS#3: Nurse, your patient is getting out of his restraints."

Triage nurse (martyr and victim): "Help!"

Complaints

The physicians meet and complain about the nurses.

The PAs meet and carry on about the nurses.

The administrators meet and want to cut the nurses.

The nurses meet and complain about each other.

Just going with the flow.

Cacophony

The phones ring incessantly. The patients groan, moan, wheeze, and curse. The stretchers squeak by. The doctors yell orders and the nurses yell back. The intercoms blare. The monitors beep. The sirens wail. The ventilators hum. The inmates' handcuffs clang against the side rails. The families complain. The babies cry.

And I try to listen to my patient's lungs.

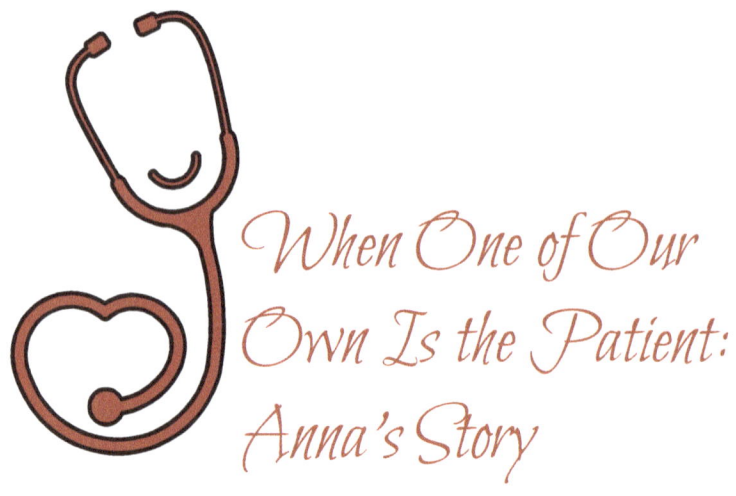

When One of Our Own Is the Patient: Anna's Story

"Trauma notification coming in"...

It was not just any other trauma patient, not just a stranger. The woman on the EMS guerney groaned in pain. Her face bloodied and disfigured, her hair matted with drying blood, the face almost beyond recognition, until I saw the nurse's uniform. Just like my own.

"Anna", I whispered her name but it sounded loud in a room suddenly rendered quiet by the shared recognition. Anna was one of the senior nurses in the ED, and she was well-loved by all of us. Even the surgeons respected her. She was the ED's toughest nurse, and we were all proud of her.

There was just one muffled curse then the trauma chief's voice spurred everyone into action. We listened as we moved Anna to the stretcher. The EMS paramedic's voice quavered with the report. "We got the call about the assault from about two streets away from the hospital. She was assaulted by her ex-husband. She's breathing and moving all extremities. She's awake, alert, and oriented but she cannot talk much because of her swollen face."

The other paramedic chimed in, "And her ex was arrested by the cops. A few construction men came to her aid, but I think they beat him up too.". I hoped that he was beaten up bad too. I was also relieved that the police did not bring that evil man to our ED.

As I cut her scrubs, I felt my eyes sting with the tears, which I had to blink away. My heart was in my throat. My hands were shaking. I locked my knees and leaned into the stretcher to prevent myself from falling. Damn it, I had to be strong because I better be the best trauma nurse there is for Anna.

I saw the fear in the staff's eyes. It was surreal to be taking care of one of our own. Anna was the trauma nurse for the day; she just went out for her lunch break and now she was lying down on the same stretcher that she just prepared.

Just like the professionals that we were, the team went to work. The other nurses looked as determined as I was as we all took our positions and did exactly what she taught us to do. Our trauma team worked in sync. The patient was one of our very own.

The ED doctors and the surgeons methodically did their assessments, Airway good, breathing on her own, no pneumothorax, vitals good. FAST was negative. As soon as the IVs were inserted, the tetanus and the antibiotics were given, we got Anna readied for the CT scans. I scooted around to her side and held her hand. Anna squeezed my hand tightly, and I said "We got you.".

As we passed through the trauma door, several hands reached out to move the stretcher, a few "I love you's from the staff" followed Anna into the CT scan. I think everybody held their breaths as we waited for the test results.

The rest of the staff returned to their own assignments, each one held their emotions in check as they braced against the onslaught of patients demanding their pain medications and complaining what took the staff too long to attend to their needs.

One of our own was hurt, I wanted to yell at the intoxicated patient who called out for more turkey sandwich. But I had to keep my mouth shut; even though my heart was aching for my friend.

The results came back. All negative except for one broken finger when Anna punched back in defense. That's our Anna. It seemed that the department heaved a collective sigh of relief. We admitted then to our ourselves that we feared the worst, and so we were all thankful and hugged each other.

Anna stayed out only for two weeks, but time was not enough to recover from the emotional trauma. Although she came back physically healthy, her heart was broken. After another month of showing up to work with a forced smile, she finally said her goodbyes. She relocated with her son to California, away from her husband who was in jail, to be with her mother and the rest of the family.

The last I heard, she was back to her old self, a no-nonsense nurse who intimidated the residents and the surgeons in her new hospital. Anna was back.

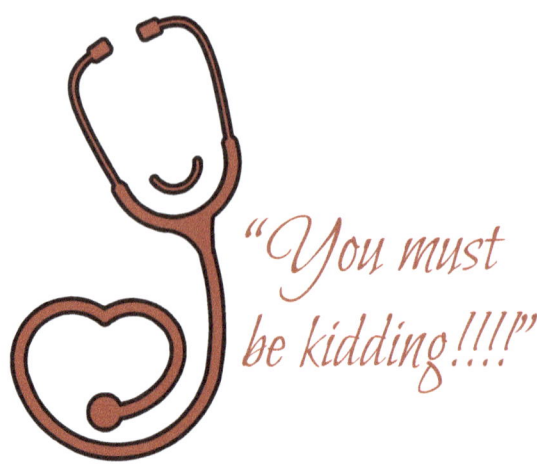

"You must be kidding!!!!"

Laughter is the best medicine, so they say. Laughter is a tonic that releases endorphins. It's a feel-good chemical, a natural high. It is an antidote to a negative vibe. A chuckle is a start to a rumbling roar of a hearty, ROFL laugh. We should always share a smile, a chuckle, a giggle, a guffaw, and a belly laugh. Negative out, positive in. Leave the work drama behind. Come and draw a cartoon.

The ER is a very funny place. There are things here that defy explanations and stories that are just too crazy to be true. But if it happened in the ER, it must be true. We don't make these things up.

A baffling case of syncope

In a case worthy of "House", some astute paramedics finally solved a baffling case of syncope.

For 3 consecutive nights at around 9pm, EMS had received a call from a wife that her husband had "fainted". The husband was often hypotensive but quickly recovered in the ER after some IV fluids. All tests came out negative and the patient was discharged in the morning, only to come back the same night. The wife stated that her husband had no physical complaints all throughout the day, but then she would find him weak and faint at night time.

On the fourth call, the EMS crew noticed the patient's bedside table. There were two tubes of medications side by side that the husband uses just before he goes to bed: one nitroglycerin ointment for the patch and one hemorrhoid ointment. The nitro medication patch on his chest to make the heart blood vessels dilate (which can lower the blood pressure too) and the Preparation-H is to relieve the pain and to reduce the swelling of the hemorrhoids.

It turns out that the patient mistakenly applies his nitro ointment to his hemorrhoids every night.

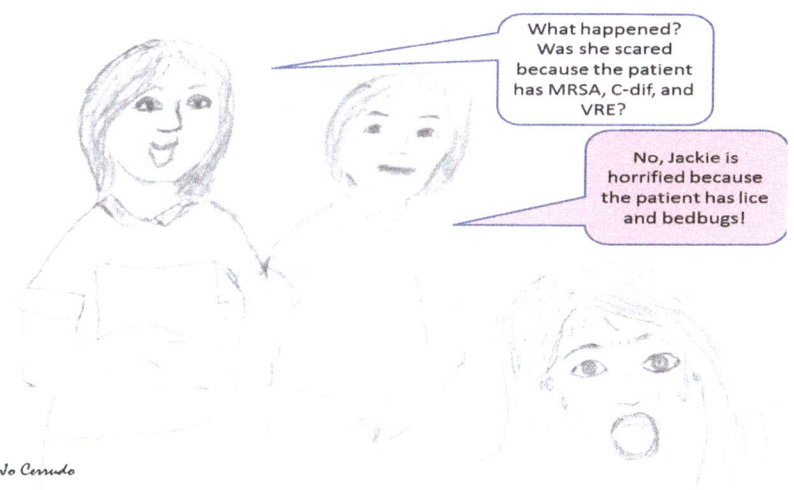

TMI

High-tech and TMI (Too Much Information) sometimes provide an awkward scene at Triage. And the nurse gets uncomfortable being shown a "selfie" without any warning. On the other hand, it is better to look at an image than having to see it in real life.

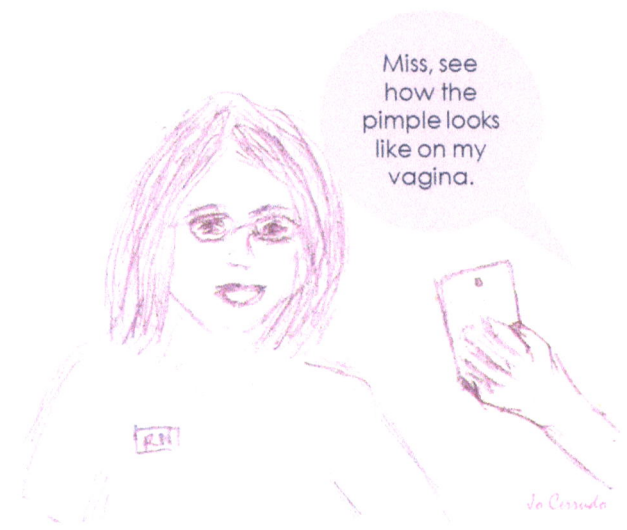

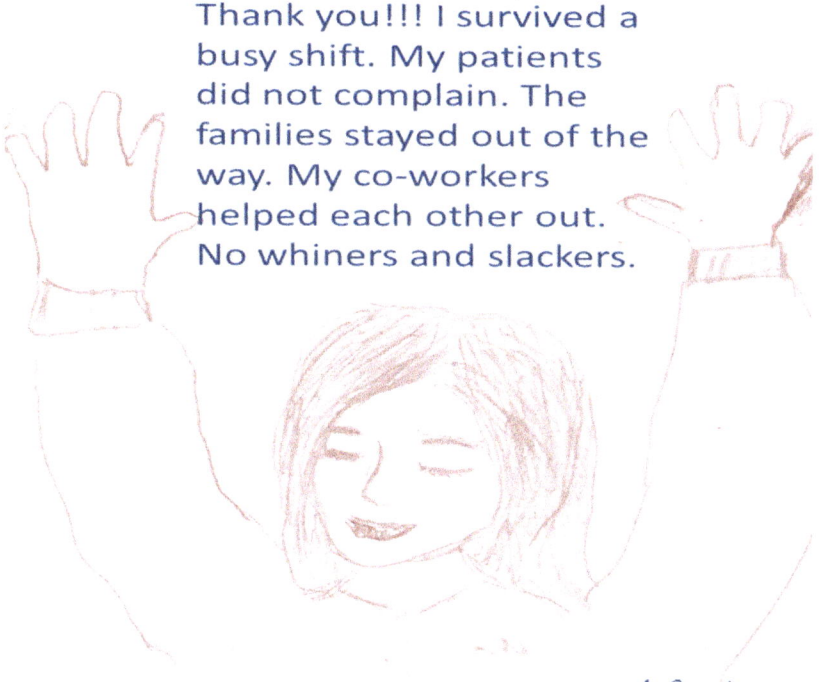

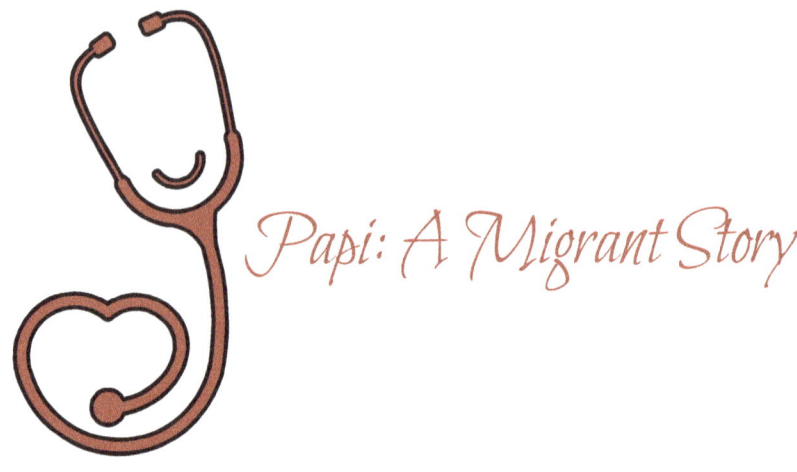

Papi: A Migrant Story

"Papi!".

The wail came from the child strapped on the EMS guerney. The Emergency Department was at its busiest with its usual din of alarms, and conversations between staff and patients, but that single word stopped me in my tracks. I could hardly see the patient with the crowd gathered around him, but I could hear the anguish and desperation from that single word. The child was shouting for his father. He was hoarse, his voice cracking.

Two men in black shirts emblazoned with the word ICE stood silent but watched everybody with eagle eyes. Their stern faces as they stood next to the patient did not invite any questions. A social worker from the detention shelter presented herself to the triage nurse. "We need a Psychiatric consult for the kid, he tried to bang his head on the floor after he was caught running away… again."

As the triage nurse reached out to put the blood pressure cuff on the boy, he cowered in fear and started screaming unintelligibly. The only word that we understood was "Papi". He repeated it over and over again, as if such repetition will conjure the man. His voice was hoarse, from hours of screaming. The social worker spoke in Spanish to the boy and tried to calm him down. The boy clung to the social worker, the person most familiar to him. His lips quivered and his beautiful brown eyes spoke of the terror he felt surrounded by strangers.

The patient was a 7-year-old from Guatemala who was separated from his father at the Immigration Center. He lost his mother two years ago from a violent attack by a drug gang in his city. Father and son were caught trying to cross the border to America, to seek asylum, anything to escape what was a living hell for them. At this moment, the boy is trapped in a nightmare that no child should ever be in.

As part of the 'zero tolerance" policy against illegal immigration, the father was whisked away to the detention center and the boy was brought into the processing center with hundreds of other migrant children, also kept apart from their parents. Countless other kids who learned early on that America is not the haven that their parents thought it would be.

The pediatrician shooed everybody from the room except for the nurse and the social worker. The ICE men stood guard outside the room. The charge nurse called for the psychiatric doctor to examine the child. Until then, the staff could only try to calm him down and prevent him from bolting out of the door. He was sitting on the bed, refusing to speak with anyone else; his arms clutching a teddy bear that the nurse gave him.

It was difficult walking away from the terrified little boy. There was nothing I can do at that moment. But I will do something to share my voice to stop this cruelty to the vulnerable victims of a xenophobic law.

I do not condone illegal immigration, but is it really necessary to separate the children from their parents? This is emotional blackmail and it hurts the kids the most. Are we risking the children's mental well-being just to enforce the rules?

How much heartache could a 7-year-old take? How did it come to this that a child is taken away from his "Papi"? How did it all came down to "zero humanity"?

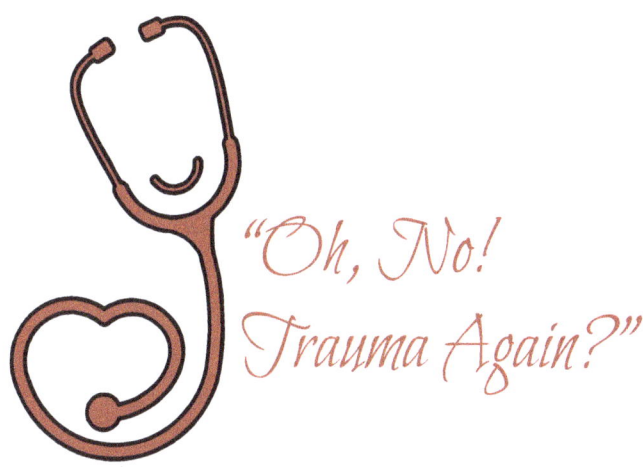

"Oh, No! Trauma Again?"

EMS notification

The red phone rings above the din of the mid-day controlled-chaos of the emergency department.

Gloria, the charge nurse sighs and picks up the phone. The resuscitation room nurses and Dr. Cooper, ED attending, approach the nursing station with expressions on their faces something akin to dread. The weariness of the back-to-back cardiac arrests and trauma cases in the past three hours is still visible on their faces. "Oh, no! Trauma again?" is the collective response from the ED staff.

Gloria writes furiously on the log book, her script almost illegible in her haste. "Stab wound to the chest, patient hypotensive 90/50, tachycardic 118, alert and responsive, paramedic, 3 minutes ETA".

The word "Trauma" is like a magic wand that transforms the frenetic atmosphere in the ED to an even more hyped-up vibe.

With a quick consultation with the ED attending, Gloria activated the Trauma Team. The phone operator repeats her every word "Trauma Level One, Adult, stab wound to the chest, Resus 1".

Team in action

The ED team galvanizes into action. Three minutes before all hell breaks loose again. The EMS notification gives them time to prepare. Sometimes, patients walk in from a trauma incident. Other times, victims from gang-related incidents are dropped off by their friends at the ambulance area. Usually, the friends scamper away when the police authorities come around to investigate.

The team leader, Dr. Cooper, calls for a brief to reinforce the roles and responsibilities of his team. There is a diagram on the wall and painted squares on the floor to remind the team. Gloria pulls one of the triage nurses to act as the scribe nurse. The team members all suit up with gowns, gloves, and goggles. The airway physician checks his airway equipment, and pulls the glide scope from the other room. The nurses prepare the chest tube set-up and the rapid infuser. The survey physician is the intern who is visibly shaking since this is his first month on the job.

Other ED staff and visitors try to come into the trauma room, only to be rebuffed by Gloria. The diminutive charge nurse is intimidating as she takes her place outside the trauma room; she will not allow any other non-essential personnel in the room. Somehow, a trauma case attracts rubber-neckers and it is Gloria's duty to do crowd control, until the nurse manager comes to take over.

The patient comes. Gloria could not help think "It's show time". The EMS paramedic directs her report to the team leader, not losing her beat as her partner motions for the transfer of the patient to the trauma stretcher. The other team members work in silence as they half-listened to the report while they undress the patient and hook him to the cardiac monitor.

The paramedic intones "This is a 20 year-old male who was involved in a battle between two gangs. He was stabbed on his right chest. The knife is with the police now. He was carrying on at the scene cursing a streak, then he became hypotensive and tachycardic so we just rushed him in here."

The ED attending glances quickly at Gloria when the paramedic mentions the gang. Gloria instinctively scans the crowd gathered outside the room. She mouths "gang activity" to the nurse manager. Marlene is an experienced ER nurse who had seen her share of gang-related traumas in her previous hospital. She immediately summons a security officer who then moves all the on-lookers away from the door. Security will need to contact NYPD to apprise them of the situation of the potential for gang retribution and to secure all entrances to the emergency department and the hospital.

The team leader asks the survey physician to report his primary assessment. "Airway is intact but there is decreased breath sound on the right. I will put a chest tube". The secondary nurse readily hands over the 38-french chest tube and insertion kit. The chest tube drains three hundred mls of blood. The

35

patient is still alert and awake but no longer belligerent. He finally realizes that he is in big trouble and he silently endures the poking from the survey physician after he received an intravenous pain medication.

Like clockwork, the nurses effortlessly insert 16-gauge IVs antecubital bilaterally. The primary nurse, Rick, hands the labeled blood tubes to Gloria who then hands them off to the patient care tech to run over to the Blood Bank. Dr. Cooper activates the massive transfusion protocol. The nurses prepare the new rapid transfuser. Gloria retrieves two units of O-negative blood from the room refrigerator.

Crowd Control

However, the responding surgeons come in droves and crowd control becomes a losing battle. Marlene tries to question everyone who responds to the trauma activation. All this talk about crowd control has to be directed to the surgeons and the consultants who bring three members of their team inside the crowded room. Everyone thinks they're indispensable.

Initially, the ED team communicated quietly with each other. The arrival of the surgeons shatters the peace, but only for a few minutes. The team leader takes control and says in a firm but controlled voice, "Everybody shut up. The only person to talk is me and the chief surgeon and the scribe nurse or whoever I ask to speak".

The scribe nurse Aysha calls out the vital signs. The blood pressure responds to the blood transfusion with the blood pressure slightly higher. "BP- 100/52, heart rate- 100". She keeps track of the vital signs and guides the survey physician as he does the secondary assessment.

The chief surgical resident discusses the patient disposition with the ED attending. He then says to his junior resident, "Call the OR now."

Case closed

Dr. Singh calls out, "Team, thank you. Our in-situ simulation is over. Please stay for a few minutes for a quick debriefing. Great job, everybody." He covers the simulation manikin and turns off the lap top with the programmed scenario.

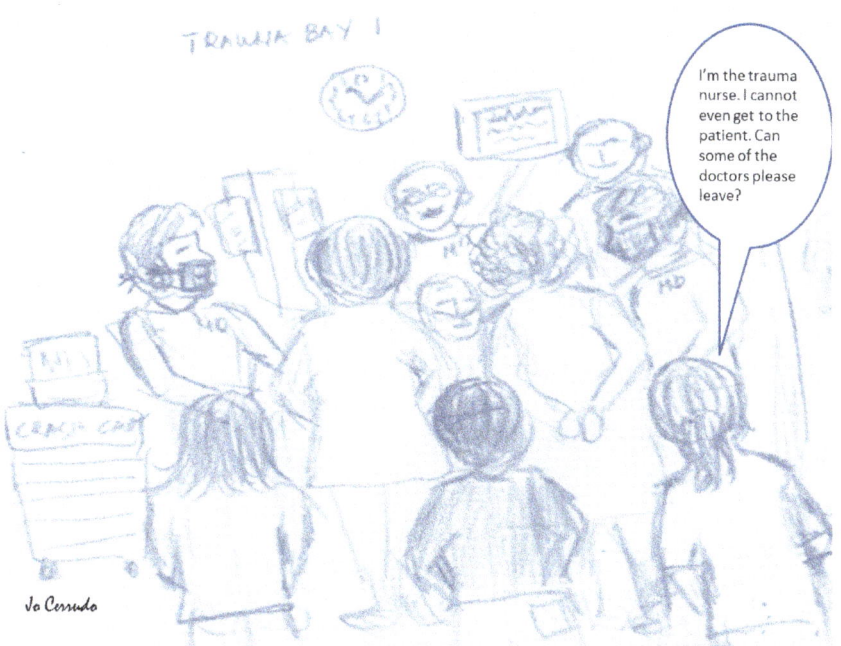

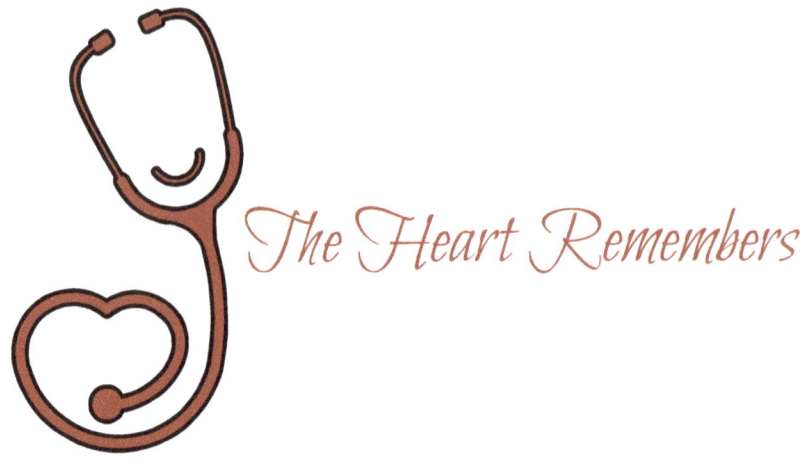

The Heart Remembers

EMS brought in an elderly man with dementia to the emergency department. The patient had become increasingly agitated due to the loud fireworks outside the nursing home. I assigned a nurses' aide to stay with the patient as we tried to sort out the bolus of patients who came in to the ED.

At the same time, a "happy drunk" staggered into the ED. Thankfully, the patient, who was a regular in the ED, just wanted an audience for his singing. The "happy drunk" entertained the triage area with opera songs like a Pavarotti. His impassioned *O Sole Mio* was surprisingly well-modulated and brought a smile to everyone, even to the ED staff who worked on the holiday, away from their family.

The elderly man stopped squirming in his stretcher. Somehow, the familiar melody broke through the cobwebs of his mind and he joined our happy drunk in total harmony. We later learned that he was an accomplished tenor in his prime. He remembered what he loved most.

I remembered the elderly man a few days ago when I

accompanied my friend Anita when she visited her mother in the nursing home. Mrs. D. sat by the window, her stares focused at the gardens outside. Was she enjoying the beautiful flowers or was she lost in her own memories? Her gnarled fingers were gently caressing the lace shawl on her lap.

My friend Anita approached her mother. "Mom, I brought my friend today."

Mrs. D. looked at us. I expected her not to recognize her daughter's friend from our apple-picking outings when we were still new in the United States. After all, she didn't even recognize her own daughter.

Alzheimer's disease had robbed Mrs. D. of her memories. She looked at her daughter like a stranger. She didn't even respond to her daughter's embrace. Her lined face was raised in fear at the sudden intrusion to her physical space.

Mrs. D. used to be a human dynamo. After she was widowed, Mrs. D. ran her daughter's home with such efficiency as her daughter and son-in-law worked hard at their careers as nurses. She was a loving but firm grandma to both of her grandkids. I remembered her humming her favorite songs whatever she was doing at that time.

Anita's family had no choice but to transfer her to a nursing home when she started wandering away from home. Mrs. D. had been missing for two days until an alert hospital worker notified the police of an unknown woman who was dropped off at the emergency department. She was lost in her own world. Mrs. D. was now a shell of her former self.

The deterioration was slow, but equally painful. What was once a vibrant woman was now profoundly changed. During the early stage of the disease, she expressed frustration for not remembering, for being a victim of her forgetfulness. Now, she looked calm, probably because she did not even realize what she was powerless to do.

Anita was sobbing in frustration. Mrs. D. was not responsive to any of her daughter's attempt at conversation. I remembered my old patient from several years ago and suggested to Anita to sing some of her mother's favorite songs.

"Saan Ka Man Naroroon" (Wherever You Are) is a Filipino love song about a woman's promise of loyalty to her loved one. This was the theme song of Anita's parents. As soon as Anita sang the song, her mother's face relaxed and her eyes focused on Anita. Mrs. D. smiled and caressed her daughter's hair.

At that moment, with the sweet melody of a beloved song, there was a respite from the darkness in her mind. Her heart remembered, even for just a few minutes.

Alzheimer's

> At that moment, with the sweet melody of a beloved song, there was a respite from the darkness in her mind. Her heart remembered, even for just a few minutes.
>
> *Jo Cerrudo*

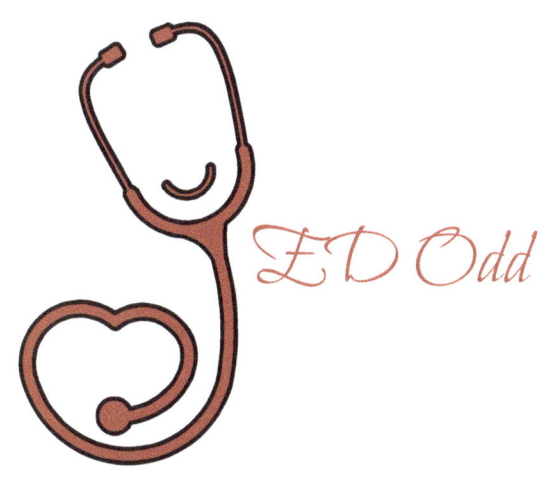

ED Odd

As if medical stories are not weird enough: Harlequin syndrome, asparagus pee smell, brain surgery via the eye socket, jeggings and yeast infection, coffee-induced strangling, steak-caused positive drug result, 'hormone of love' or 'cuddle chemical', and "sphenopalatine ganglioneuralgia" or brain freeze.

And now, Botox to cure vaginismus? I guess smoothing wrinkles takes a whole new dimension, huh?

Truth is stranger than fiction, and it has never become truer than in the ED.

Patient: "An animal went into my ear, it's now in my brain."

Doctor: "What kind of animal will go inside your brain?"

Patient: "You're rude. My left brain does not want to talk to you."

Doctor: "Can you tell your right brain to talk to me?"

At triage...

Patient: "I looked at the mirror and saw a blinking eye on my left butt."

The nurse thought the patient was crazy, but the patient insisted in being examined.

So the nurse and the intern took the patient to the room and looked at the patient's butt in question.

An eye blinked at them. On a trip to South America, an insect had burrowed itself on the patient's butt.

It's important to follow directions.

A patient bought an over-the-counter topical genital enhancement product from a neighborhood store. He did not follow directions. Instead of just rubbing the ointment, he ingested two doses in preparation for a date. He did not know that the Atropine effects would make him very, very sick.

He died the day after.

Toxic Sock Syndrome

When your patient's socks had melted into the skin, and the smell travels all the way to the hospital lobby. The patient is oblivious to the suffering around him. The staff tries to hold their breaths and waits anxiously for their shift to end.

Toxic Tampon syndrome

When a first-time user thought the tampon will absorb on its own.

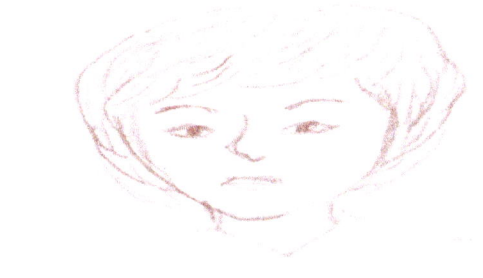

Dear patient,
Please do not experiment. EMLA is used as a numbing ointment when we start IVS on our pediatric patients. It is not a vaginal lubricant. That is why you've fainted.

Jo Corrado

**Foreign body in rectum.
All types, all sizes.**

Whatever you see, do not let the
patient see how you really feel.

Jocelyn Cerrudo Sese

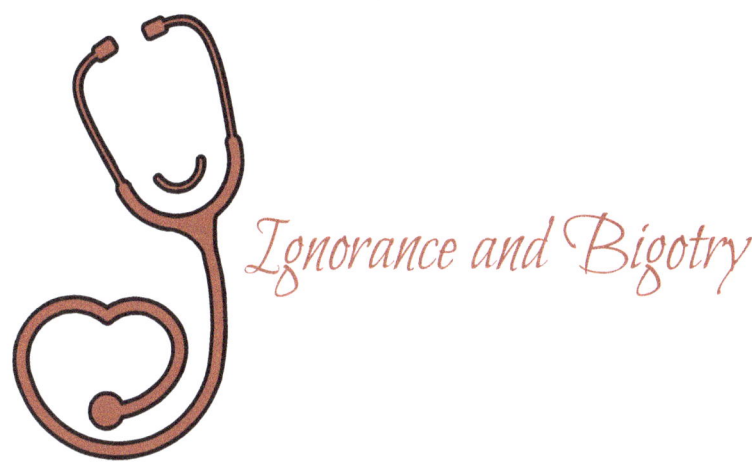

Ignorance and Bigotry

I wrote this letter about 15 years ago. Sadly, this still holds true. Somehow, the hateful vitriol is further emboldened by xenophobic rhetorics from bullies and haters. I have always worked with an exemplary diverse staff who see patients as human beings. I stand proud as an American citizen and as a nurse, even as we face all these challenges with professionalism and decency.

Dear patient,

I wish I can erase that hatred in your heart, that xenophobic attitude against anyone who doesn't look like you. You cursed at me and told me to "return to my country", even as I was just trying to take care of you. I swallowed the bile in my throat as you ranted about immigrants who stole your job. I have two college degrees, dear patient. Based on your incoherent and ungrammatical ramblings, I am pretty sure you could not perform my job.

I knew you were sick so I ignored your blatant racism. If you weren't sick, I would have insisted on behavioral limitations. I knew you were not just having a bad day, but that you had an evil heart. In your previous visit, you smacked one of my techs just for being late in bringing your meal tray.

But you were obviously sick. Your ashen complexion and your ragged breathing convinced me to ignore your rants. I allowed my orientee to interview you just so I can get enough information why you have tachycardia and back pains. I did not call security to escort you out because I realized that you needed medical help, despite the obscene gestures. You are an ignorant and a bigot, but you are my patient.

You don't know that I was the one who recognized that you were dying. You even refused to be seen by our Asian ED doctor and the African-American resident. But then, you collapsed in front of us. You don't know that I was the only one who could insert a good IV line in your fragile veins. Now that you are unconscious, you would never realize that the emergency team who took care of you was a diverse group, a multi-colored group of professionals. If you knew you were dying, would you have accepted our ministrations?

The rainbow of ethnicities in our emergency team did not divide us but instead united us in our efforts to serve the diverse community. Our team of doctors, nurses, and other ancillary staff did not care about the color of your skin. There was no question about your sexual orientation, or political and religious affiliations. All we were concerned was to race against time to save your life.

You are our patient. If you are conscious, we would not tolerate your disgusting behavior. But unfortunately, you are now intubated and brain-dead. So we have to be blind to your faults. We will not respond in kind to your ignorance and bigotry. Despite your evil thoughts, we will remain true to our sworn oath to take care of you, as we do with all our patients. I see you as a human being. No matter what.

Your Filipino-American nurse

P.S. You signed an Organ Donor Card. It is great that you did not state a preference for the recipients of your organs. I'm sorry that you would not be able to read this letter. I was hoping this would open your eyes and touch your heart.

I DON'T CARE IF YOU'RE BLACK, WHITE, ASIAN, UGLY, PRETTY, GAY, STRAIGHT, JEWISH, CATHOLIC, OR AGNOSTIC.

If you're a patient, I will take care of you.

Just. Don't. Hit.

Jocelyn Cerrudo Sese

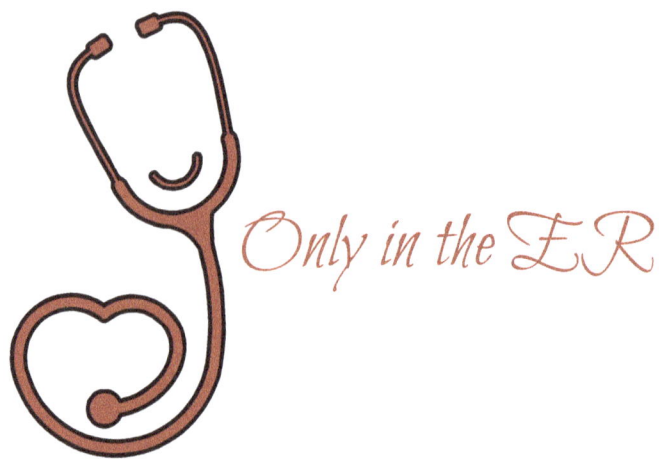

Only in the ER

The nurse instructed the patient to undress and to provide a urine specimen. She handed the patient a clothing bag and a specimen container. Minutes later, he handed the nurse the clothing bag with a dark amber colored fluid in it. He reasoned out that the specimen container was too small to hold all his urine.

Whenever I come out into the ED Waiting Room to call a patient, I always feel like a celebrity. Patients and families rush up to me like I'm a goddess who's going to sweep them into the examination rooms. Right! Don't they know that the ER is like a madhouse and that it's almost Standing Room only?

Sometimes I feel like the hungry crowd is closing in on me. I can feel their hot breaths of anticipation and see the hostile glances from those who are left behind.

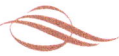

The EMS is between a rock and a hard place. Because of the EMTALA/COBRA laws, NY EMS cannot refuse transports for the following:

1. "I have a clinic appointment and I can't afford a taxi."
2. "I didn't make it to the Methadone clinic before closing time. I need to go to the hospital for my dose."
3. "It's too cold out in the streets and I don't want to stay in the shelter. Bring me to the hospital."
4. "I just wanna talk with somebody."

Sometimes at triage, it's like pulling teeth just to get the right information from the patient. They either bring all their chronic complaints, or they expect you to deduce their medical history from their medication bottles.

Then, after all that, their complaints change when they see the physicians.

Most alcoholics are Houdinis. They can get out of the fanciest restraints. One advice I've followed through the years: Undress these patients and keep their clothes inaccessible. And if they do get out of restraints, it's easier to catch them. Just follow the ones running naked through the ER.

Overheard at Triage, in the middle of the blizzard...

Patient 1: "I have ingrown toe-nail.'

Patient 2: "So what if I have this arm pain for 15 years?"

Patient 3: "I need a sonogram, my head is buzzing."

Patient 4: "Is lunch served yet?"

Patient 5: "I have itching down there. Do you want to see?"

Patient 6: "I need a physical."

Patient 7: " Is Psych open?"

Nurse: "Oh yes, they still have room for one more patient."

When undressing a patient for exam, be ready for the barrage of scents that assault the senses and challenge your gut. Don't remove the socks unless absolutely necessary.

Sometimes, my ears ring because of the constant onslaught of curses from patients and families. I handle them as firm and as professional as I can be. And in my mind, I curse them back in my own language. It helps.

A doctor looks around wearily, "Who's my nurse?"

I ask him back, "It's 12:00 o'clock already, don't you know who your nurses are?"

For the umpteenth time, I had to explain to the irate relative. "Sorry, sir, there's a lot of patients today. Many much sicker than your wife. Yes, we know that her ingrown toenail is hurting too much."

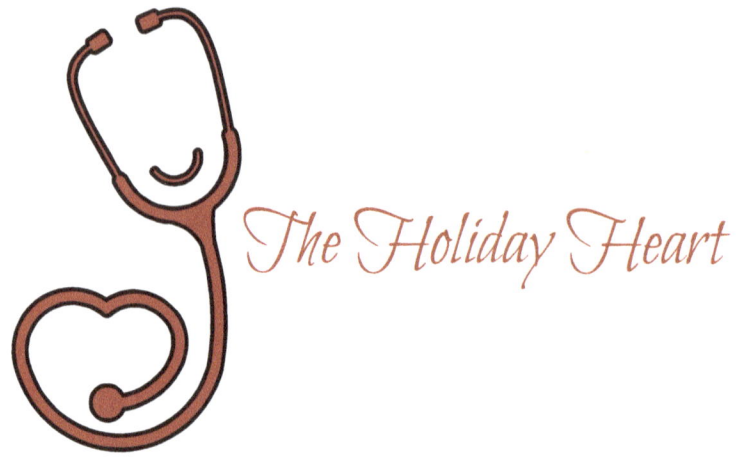

The Holiday Heart

During the holiday season when families spend time together, someone out there is looking for some love and attention. Like the woman from Oklahoma who posted on Craigslist "Anybody need a grandma for Christmas? I'll even bring food and gifts for the kids! I have nobody and it really hurts." This post went viral and illustrated the stark reality that many of our elderly population are isolated from their families. Actually, not just the elderly; there are many lonely people in the world.

In the merriment of the holiday season, hospitals see a lot of patients overcome with depression. Those who are medically sick sometimes spend the holidays with the staff who had to leave their families to take care of their patients. In the emergency department, we continue to get patients who choose to binge-drink to fight their loneliness and ended up with Holiday Heart syndrome.

One New Year's eve several years ago, I stayed with one lonely 70 y/o patient as we watched on tv for the Times Square crystal ball to drop. She was waiting for her family to pick her up. She was teary-eyed, confused at the babble of voices in our crowded ED, unable to understand the language. But she smiled when I brought her food and counted down with her during the ball drop. As I hugged her, I was reminded of my mom, miles away in the Philippines. The patient eased my homesickness as I comforted her. Mrs. Chen bowed to me and said "Xie-xie" (Thank you in Mandarin).

Thank you to all of those who work during the holidays. At a time when all others celebrate the holidays in the comfort of their homes with their loved ones, it is a blessing to bring some kind of comfort and peace to those who need them the most. During the holidays, the ED is not always crowded so there is always a chance to spread some cheer around. A little touch, a little smile, and some time to just listen go a long way to ease a lonely heart.

Holiday Heart Syndrome

In 1978, Philip Ettinger described "Holiday heart syndrome" (HHS) for the first time, as the occurrence, in healthy people without heart disease known to cause arrhythmia, of an acute cardiac rhythm disturbance, most frequently atrial fibrillation, after binge drinking. The name is derived from the fact that episodes were initially observed more frequently after weekends or public holidays.

https://www.ncbi.nlm.nih.gov/pmc/articles/PMC3998158/

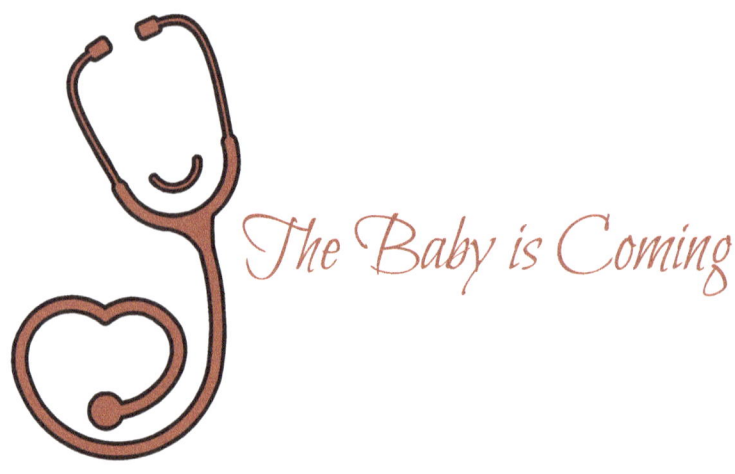

The Baby is Coming

Some babies could not wait to enter the world. They could not wait for their mother to reach the Labor and Delivery Room. I guess if you have to go, you gotta go.

I have seen so many babies delivered in the ER. For some reason, some people still admonish the mothers, "No puje! Don't push!". As if you can fight Mother Nature.

An impending birth is always an exciting event in the ER. We see so many sad cases, so many deaths, so a baby's wail in the midst of an intoxicated patient's rants is always a welcome sound. There's nothing like a new life to reaffirm our purpose in being.

I helped deliver a baby in a cab outside the ED. The mother grunted then yelled at her husband for making her pregnant again. It was Baby number 5.

One time, I saw the patient's spandex began to sag at the crotch. I dove to catch the baby before it slid down on the floor.

Another time, I followed a teenager to the bathroom, just because I was suspecting that she was not just carrying belly fat. When she screamed, I fished the baby out of the toilet. The beautiful baby girl crunched her face, and cried. It was the most glorious wail I ever heard (except for my own son's triumphant cry to the world).

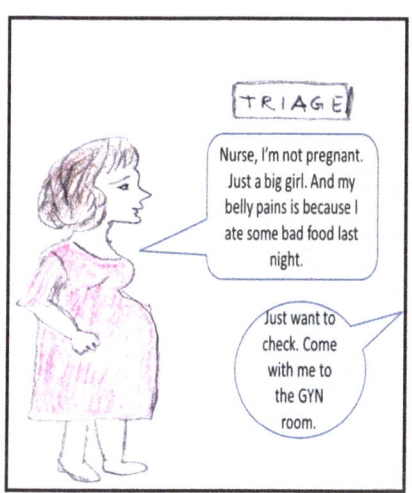
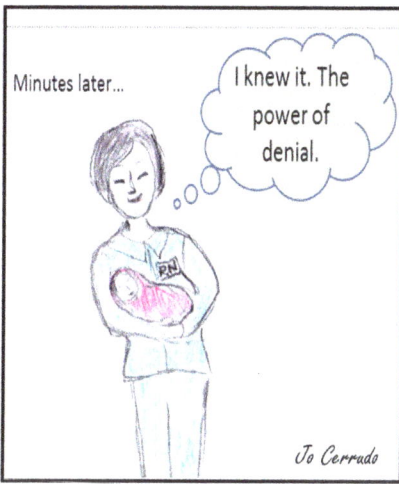

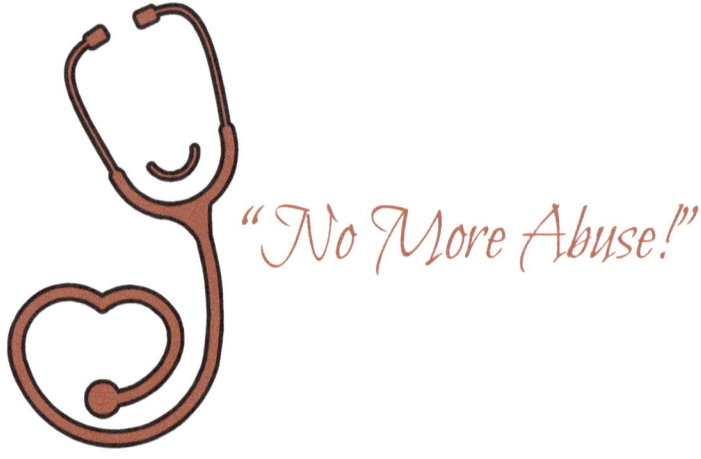

"No More Abuse!"

The 18-year-old woman sat quietly on the bed. Her face bore the bruises that could not be hidden any much longer. The abuse from her much-older husband had escalated.

I remembered her from a month ago when she came in with a twisted ankle and bruises on her arm. She said she fell down the stairs. The triage nurse suspected domestic violence but the patient vehemently denied it. Her husband came rushing into the ER, distraught that his wife's care was not expedited enough. He stated that he was a lawyer and will sue the hospital if his wife did not get the best of care.

Now, she sat in her chair, her back rigid, and her eyes closed as she waited for the detective to finish his conversation with the social worker. As I waited by the door to come in to her room, I noticed the rivulet of tears running down her battered face.

The mother-in-law was as demanding as the husband. She was horrified that her son is being accused to be a wife-beater. "My son is a partner in his law firm". As if that was some valid reason to use his wife as his punching bag. As if being a successful professional excused him to abuse his wife. Security escorted the husband and mother-in-law out of the ER for disruptive behavior.

The wife was an immigrant from another country, sponsored by her husband on spousal visa. She was unable to stand up to her husband, bound by her custom of obedience, crippled by her financial dependence on the man who controlled the purse strings, and who hid her passport.

She was a beautiful woman, her hair lustrous and her face unlined, but her eyes showed defeat and hopelessness. She said her father will not accept her back in her country. The blame was laid on her head for failure to serve her husband as what a dutiful wife should do. She straightened up and forcefully said, "I cannot take the abuse anymore. No more abuse!".

The social worker came back into the room with great news. They were able to contact the patient's sister in Florida. She was in the same situation five years ago, but had successfully left her husband, and built a new life far away with her kids. She wanted her sister to fly to Florida.

The detective also informed us that the patient's husband is now under arrest. He handed the patient her passport. She smiled, and her eyes shone with hope.

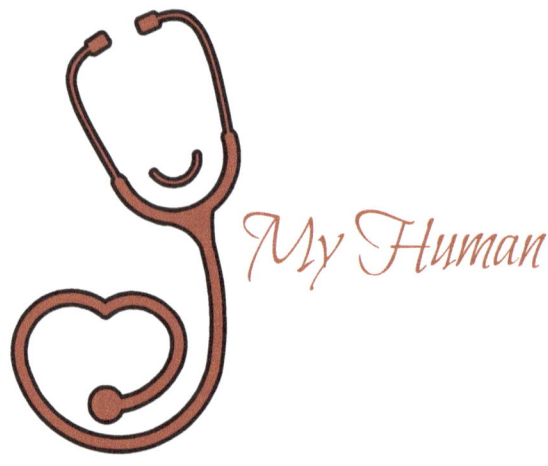

My Human

Written from the perspective of a service animal

I am a service animal. My human is who I am loyal to. Please do not make fun of him because he is disabled. He is trying to make the most of what he's got. I am the only one who can understand him. I go with him everywhere, even to the hospitals. As long as I behave, I can stay at the bedside.

I am his seeing eye dog. He can see shapes with his right eye. He lost his left eye several years ago in Afghanistan. As he walks by my side, he feels for the tug of my leash to warn him of danger in the path ahead. He responds to my subtle moves. Step to the left, step to the right. When I stop, he stops. After four years together, he trusts me. I once saved us both when I warned him of a car who whizzed by without regard to the blind man and his dog.

Yesterday, my human had to go to the hospital. The security officer tried to block me from coming into the emergency department and wanted me chained to a corner. I did not growl at him, but I was tempted to. It's good that the nurse came right on time to lecture the security officer of my human's rights.

I guess the officer was just too eager. There are a few people who try to pass off their pets as service animal. If the dog is just for emotional support, that is not enough to qualify as a service dog. My human told me of Mrs. Harris, our next-door neighbor, who tried to smuggle Rosita into the hospital. That chihuahua could not stay quiet at all. She even tried to bite the nurse. Ahem, then there is Senor Diaz. His pet ferret is not a service animal but he still claims he needs Chester for emotional support.

My human suffers from what he calls PTSD. When there are these loud things in the distance that he calls "damn fireworks", he cowers in the corner, just like me. We hold each other, and I try to calm myself so that he can stop shaking.

My human said that the American with Disabilities Act protects his rights as a disabled person. The public cannot discriminate against a person with a disability. He said that nobody can demand proof that I am a service dog especially since it's obvious that he is disabled. I don't have to have a license or a certificate. Sometimes, I wear my special vest except during the hot summer months.

When my human meets up with his old friends from his old platoon, that is when I also bond with the other service dogs. One German shepherd barks when his human's blood sugar is getting low. A golden Labrador warns his human before he gets a seizure. I am a beagle and I am the most experienced dog in my group.

Oh, have you heard that miniature horses can also serve as service animals? I would love to meet one someday. Two years ago, an artist was prevented from boarding a United Airlines flight with her "emotional support" animal. Not a dog or a miniature pony as allowed by the American Disabilities Act. She tried to bring a PEACOCK on the plane. Really?

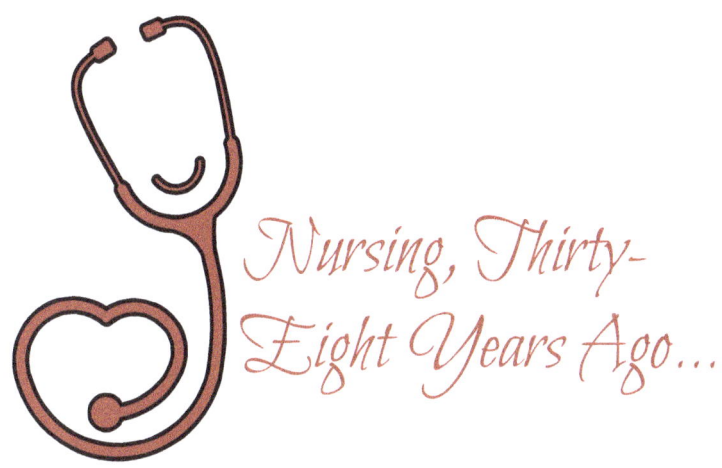

Nursing, Thirty-Eight Years Ago...

Thirty-eight years ago, long before I started my ER nursing career, I stepped into Coler Memorial Hospital on a cold January morning. Coler Hospital is/was one of two chronic care hospitals specializing in rehabilitative care (the other one is Goldwater Hospital) located on Roosevelt Island.

Our group of young Filipino nurses newly-flown to New York was culture-shocked. I thought that our patients spoke with difficult accents, all slangs yet full of grammatical errors. I was convinced that the doctors misspelled their orders and were insulted when we questioned duplicate medications.

Our nursing supervisors towered over us with doubt written on their faces. They probably were wondering how these naïve, young women could stand up to the bossy LPNs who used to rule the roost. We were usurpers to the throne. We didn't know any better and how dare we come to this place expecting to find our way into their nursing world.

But dared we did. We held our own, learned the slang, and worked our way to earn the respect. Not only of our supervisors, but mostly by our patients who delighted in our enthusiasm and compassion. My supervisor used to challenge me to go beyond my comfort zone. Somehow the patients who were abandoned to our care became our own grandparents. We held their hands and listened to their nostalgic remembrances of lives spent caring for their loved ones. We dried their tears just as we dried our own tears of loneliness for families left behind in the Philippines.

"You're my favorite, Cerrudo.", one of the chronic dialysis patients rewarded me with this one day. I quickly bragged to my friends about how I finally won over the most difficult patient in the unit. My friends did not even give me time to relish my victory; She told them the same thing last week. I was Sessa's favorite that time because I slipped her an extra ice cream.

My first unit was the Medical ICU. One part was the chronic ventilator unit where patients remained attached to ventilators; we became experts with trache care, suctioning, and communicating with our patients the best way we could.

Mr. Alston used to clench his jaw and blink his eyes three times if he wanted things done. One bedridden patient could only give a lop-sided smile if we positioned him right. Mrs. Richards frowned if we didn't tuck her bedsheets right and gave us thumbs up when we did. Young Alli smiled at everything we did for her, as we wiped the drool on her neck, cleaned her trache and brushed the tangles on her hair. I massaged the contracted feet of my ALS patient who continued to have a vibrant mind while his body wasted away.

The patients were our family… and every time one passed

away, we cried with the rest of the staff. Most of the time, the nurses were the only ones who grieved their passing because the families had long abandoned them.

Two years later, I was promoted to a head nurse position in a general med-surg unit with 40 patients. I took my share of duties as part of functional nursing. There was usually one medication nurse who starts and finishes the day giving meds with printed medication cards; from back to the front of the unit where meds were given thru gastrostomy tubes. Another nurse and I worked with a group of two nurses' aides as we fed, bathed, exercised, and walked the patients. At 3pm, we started our narrative charting, our notes the same every day except for the vital signs and whether patients had bowel movement or not.

Thankfully, the technology and staffing got much better. The suction EKG bulbs were horrendous, and left their distinct marks on our patients' frail chests, the yucky gel too difficult to clean off. The manual mercury sphygmomanometer is now a thing of the past. Now it's just a button to push on the automatic cardiac monitor and we get a veritable riches of data: BP, HR, oxygen saturation, MAP, endtidal CO2.

Gone are the medication cards, those 2 by 2 index cards with hand-written transcription of medication orders, the dosage times written in black, green, and red. Gone are the Kardexes with nursing diagnoses that never changed. Gone are the hand-written doctor's orders that were meant to confuse.

Back then, I was new, nervous, and unsure of my place in this world. I left the hospital years later to start my career in ER nursing. Along the way, I learned valuable lessons that have served me well in my profession. That the rewards of nursing far exceed the material blessings. That the compassion I have shown my patients was the greatest gift I could have given them.

When the patient needs a hand, it doesn't matter if the hand that is offered is that of a baby boomer or a millennial. At the end of the day, the patients will remember a nurse who gave them the respect that they deserve.

Through the nurses I teach, I wish that a compassionate nurse lives on.

EKG suction bulbs... the way we were.

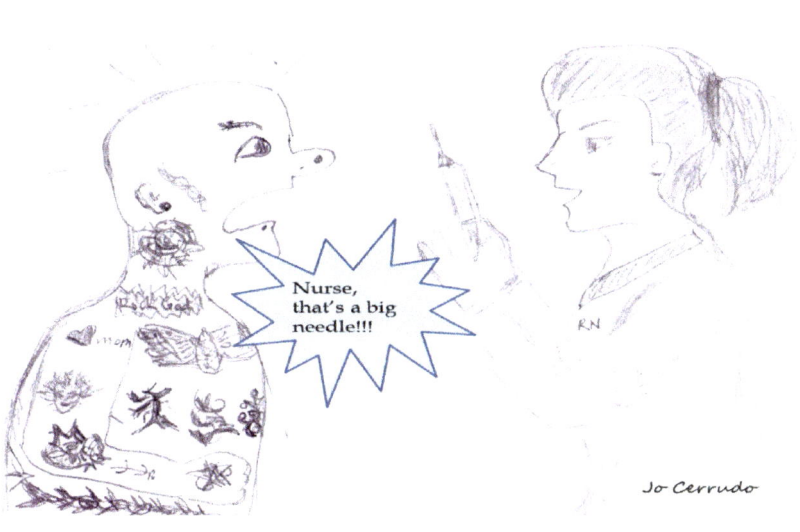

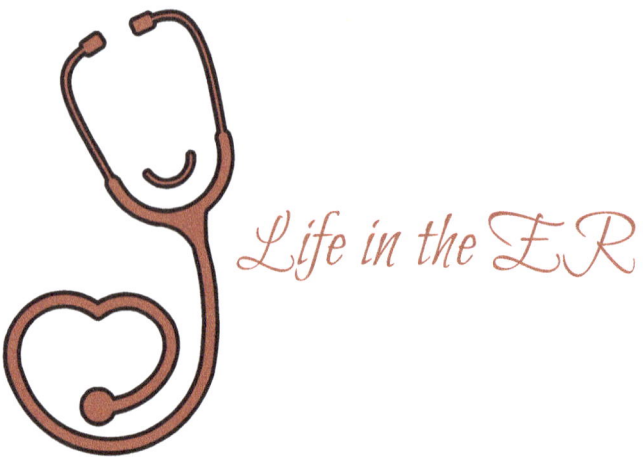

Life in the ER

"Oh, what a beautiful morning. Oh, what a beautiful day", sang this 250-lb flushed-face, alcohol-reeking man who graced our ED one day. He was a happy drunk, winking at the nurses, and even trying to slap a female clerk's behind as she passed. After we restrained him up, and pushed him into a private room, he stopped singing. He was silent, but not for long.

Out he came, walked out of the room, buck naked, with the stretcher still strapped on his back.

What's worse than a hypochondriac patient?

A gullible nurse.

Life in the ER

Superstitions in the ED:

1. Do not ever say the "Q" word.
2. Cardiac arrests come in threes.
3. Full Moon brings in patients.

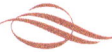

She looked haggard, walked like a Zombie, and snapped at everybody. Beware the Burned-out-nurse. Time for a vacation again.

Before the ED had our electronic documentation, patients sign up on a paper form. Liz, the triage nurse, loudly called for the next name... "Culo Grande, Culo Grande". Nobody responded, and instead most of the patients were grinning, some with chests heaving with laughter every time Liz called out the name.

A Hispanic hospital police officer sidled up to Liz, "Do you know what 'Culo Grande' means?" It means "Big Ass.".

Liz refused to triage after that.

My non-medical friend asked, "How come when you nurses get together, you take so much pleasure in grossing each other out with talk about the hospital? Imagine talking about these fluids during meals. Yuck!"

A friend dropped by one day when the ER was in gridlock. It was 12 noon and the EMS stretchers were lined up all the way down to the ER ambulance door. Patients were cursing, and telephones were ringing. Nurses and doctors rushed through the crowded corridors to respond to a Trauma Team call.

With such disbelief in her face, she gasped, "You must be crazy to work here."

The staff around us chorused, "We all are!".

Everybody knows CG, our resident drunk. He came via EMS, he came walking, he came in any which way he can especially on cold winter nights. He slipped in and out of the ER in sync with our mealtimes. Then he was gone for a month.

He came back one day, all cleaned up, dressed up in clean dress pants and shirt and a blazer. His sister got him into Rehab. We patted him on the back, even high-fived with him. "Way to go.", "Keep it up". TL smiled ear-to-ear, and blushed beet-red as he accepted all the compliments from the staff. We all felt that there was still hope in life.

A month later, he came back drunk and seizing.

Life in the ER

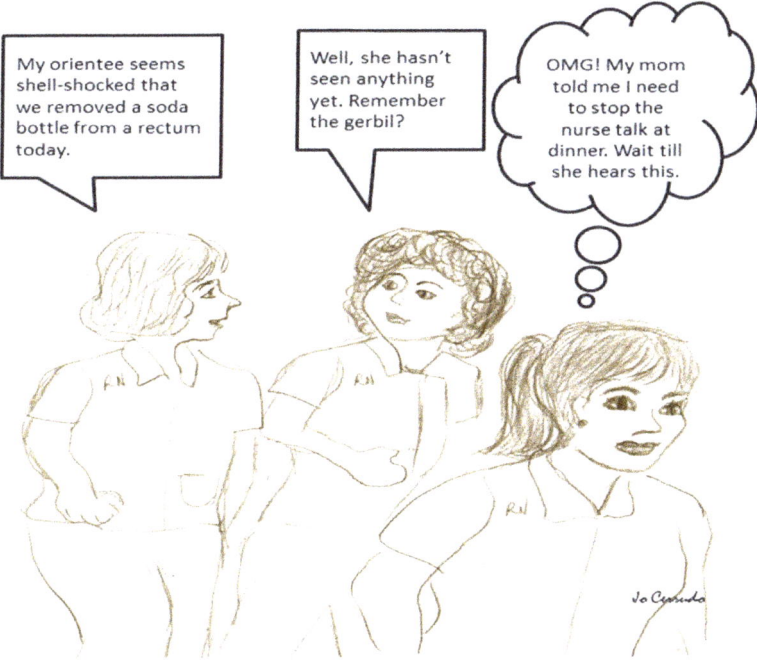

The red EMS notification phone rings. All ED personnel stopped in their tracks and listened with bated breath. The triage nurse answers, "No, sir, this is not a pizza parlor."

Everybody gasped. On the endoscopy machine screen, the patient's stomach lining was littered with debris of her experiments with exotic food: an eraser, a paper clip, a teaspoon, a capped syringe, and a ring.

The GI consultant exclaimed, "So, that's where my wedding ring went!".

The medical intern volunteered to do the chest compressions during a code. The strong, even strokes reflected on the defibrillator screen. Then the compressions became weaker, slower until the intern dropped on the floor.

Somebody said, "Uh-oh, there's still Nitropaste on the patient's chest."

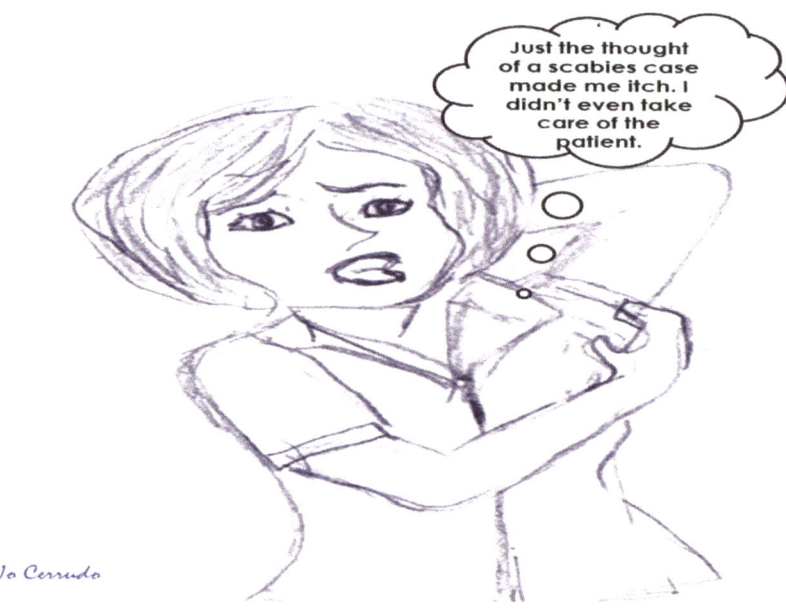

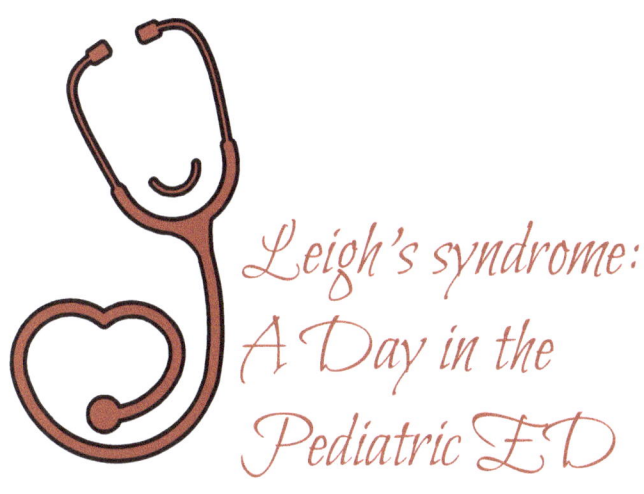

Leigh's syndrome: A Day in the Pediatric ED

It was an EMS notification of a 2-year-old in cardiac arrest that stopped us in our tracks. The Pediatric ED was unusually quiet that morning when the EMS call came. Our hearts did a collective thump when we got the call.

Some of the adult ED nurses rushed to the Peds ED to help. The rest of the ED staff called their families to check on their kids.

The resuscitation room was crowded with personnel, four nurses, three doctors and a respiratory therapist. All trying to change destiny.

This poor boy should not die, too soon, too young, I thought. Did he choke on something; does he have a congenital disease? Kids are not supposed to come in cardiac arrest.

From what I could see from my vantage point, he had thick hair and long-lashed eyes. His eyes were thankfully closed. A beautiful Indian baby face. The EMS had already intubated him at home, scooped him up from his crib, and brought him to our hospital.

One of the nurses kept his rhythm as he maintained a one-hand compression on the child's sternum. The senior pediatric nurse's face was wet with unchecked tears. The pediatric attending's brow was creased in concentration as he managed the resuscitation efforts. Another nurse was checking the Braslow tape to guide with the medication doses.

The cardiac monitor showed asystole. The orders came rushing: Epinephrine, continue CPR, Sodium bicarb, warmer, saline bolus, anything.

"He has Leigh's syndrome.". The resident informed the team after he got this information from the mother. Everyone's shoulders sagged with the news.

Leigh's syndrome is a rare neurological disorder that progresses rapidly in mental and psychomotor abilities, and eventually respiratory failure. It is a death sentence, just like some of the other congenital diseases that are brought to the PEDS ED every day.

The triage nurse had escorted the mother to the next room while the doctors and nurses worked on her baby. There was nothing to do, but just sit with her as she closed her eyes in prayer. Her hands were on her mouth, as if she was trying not to break into hysterical tears; clinging to the hope that her son will survive.

I relieved the triage nurse from her vigil with the mother. Her bleak eyes glistened as she looked hopefully for any information about her son. I could only say, "They're still taking care of your son."

The mother's sari looked big on her; she must have just grabbed whatever she could. Her husband was just on his way in. The charge nurse gave instructions for the taxi driver-husband to just park at the ambulance ramp immediately.

Her soft voice was tinged with worry. "He was just seen by the doctor two days ago, and he was doing well. He was sleeping two hours ago. Then when I looked at him, he was not breathing at all"... her voice trailed away as she stifled a sob.

Even in the face of certain death, the PEDS staff would not give up, but all their efforts were unsuccessful. It seemed so much longer but it was just thirty minutes. At the end, the baby was pronounced dead.

After the doctor broke the news to the parents, the mother rushed to her son's bed. From the room, we heard the plaintive keening of a grieving mother. The mother's cries tore into our hearts, and even the paramedics were dabbing their eyes. The sound of sorrow stays with you for a long time.

"This breaks my heart every time.", the seasoned pediatric nurse told me.

"I'm glad you're here because I would not know how to deal with this heart break.", I said to her. I was being truthful. Pediatrics had always scared me.

Emergency nurses are supposed to be the tough guys, but in my opinion, the nurses from Pediatrics, Oncology, and the Hospice are the toughest of them all.

And in our ER, there was no time to dwell on that heart-wrenching scene. Just an hour later, a febrile baby came in and was worked up for sepsis. She lived.

Just a few hours later, five kids were pulled out from their burning house. The fire started in the kitchen, but thankfully, all the kids (siblings and cousins) were fine, especially after an enterprising social worker brought in some lollipops. No smoke inhalation, no skin burns.

The Pediatric ED staff does an incredible job every day, and as the nurse said, "It's never easy to lose a child, even when it's not our own."

Leigh's disease is a rare inherited neurometabolic disorder that affects the central nervous system in infants between the ages of three months and two years. Leigh's disease can be caused by mutations in mitochondrial DNA or by deficiencies of an enzyme called pyruvate dehydrogenase. Symptoms of Leigh's disease usually progress rapidly. The earliest signs may be poor sucking ability, and the loss of head control and motor skills. These symptoms may be accompanied by loss of appetite, vomiting, irritability, continuous crying, and seizures. As the disorder progresses, symptoms may also include generalized weakness, lack of muscle tone, and episodes of lactic acidosis, which can lead toimpairment of respiratory and kidney function.

https://rarediseases.org/rare-diseases/leigh-syndrome/

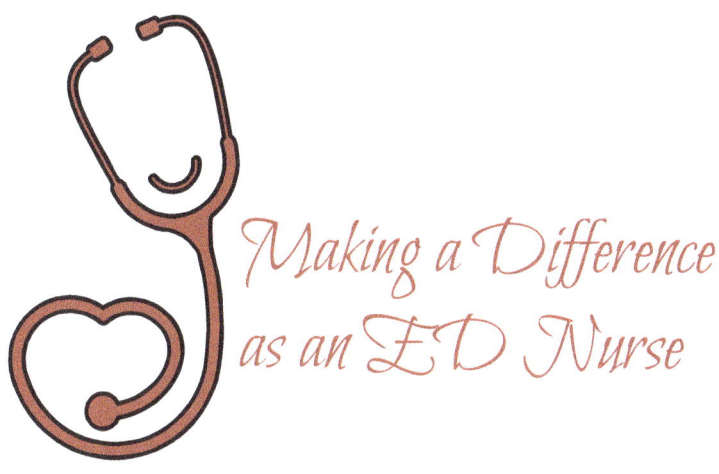

Making a Difference as an ED Nurse

As a STAFF NURSE in the Emergency Department, I made a difference when...

- I was the IV nurse to go to for the smallest and difficult-to-access veins, long before those fancy vein-finder devices ever made it to production

- I volunteered to work another shift of overtime, even after a few hours of sleep from partying with friends

- I could last longer doing CPR than some of my co-workers who huffed and puffed after just three cycles

- I sang and danced to calm down a Down syndrome patient who was having a meltdown in the midst of a noisy ER

- I multi-tasked to cover another nurse who needed a little time to recover from a bad trauma case

- I helped out a tech who was busy elsewhere and did

- the EKG myself for a patient with atypical presentation of chest pain (she actually had a heart attack)

- I intervened to prevent a fight between two intoxicated patients (I was almost hit by an errant left hook)

- I cross-checked the new nurse's drug calculations and prevented a medication error.

- I triaged a quiet, stoic elderly man who sat patiently for his turn before a loud, obnoxious female who complained of having an asthma attack (while speaking in full sentences and clutching a bag of chips). He turned out to be in sepsis.

- I held my dying patient's hand so he didn't die alone.

And many more to mention…. I miss those good ole days.

As a NURSE EDUCATOR in the Emergency Department, I made a difference when…

- I taught the nurses how to triage, to use across-the-room-assessments, and to trust their instinct, and to not be intimidated when the doctors questioned their judgments.

- I watched like a hawk and did not let the nurses pass competency until they can demonstrate setting up chest tubes and rapid infusers to my satisfaction

- I failed a nurse's orientation because she did not meet her milestones, but most especially, she had the nastiest attitude towards her patients.

- I patiently counseled an earnest novice nurse who had the potential to become better, but just needed a little guidance to boost her self-esteem

- I taught the nurses how to read the EKG and "saw" the "light bulb" in my students' eyes

- I gave feedback with respect

- I challenged the nurses' minds so they would not accept old processes just because they're used to doing them

- I encouraged the nurses' aides and techs to study for their nursing degree

- I engaged my students in my class to participate in robust discussions

- I prepared specialty certification materials for the nurses and pushed them to go for advanced degrees.

I felt validated when I meet former students/nurses who told me that they learned so much from me.

As a NURSE LEADER in the Emergency Department, I made a difference when...

- I closed the vacancy gaps and improved the unit's staffing

- I promoted nurse engagement, to improve retention and satisfaction so they feel proud of being part of the work family

- I collaborated with interdisciplinary staff to improve unit processes and patient workflow

- I managed my budget but will always choose patient safety over not approving for overtime when the ED is in surge

- I managed up or acknowledged the staff when they were doing great or when they caught a near-miss or potential error).

- I will always find a way to nominate them for a Nurse Excellence Award or for a DAISY.

- I encouraged advancement in the nurses' practice by using evidence-based care

- I practiced Just Culture when staff makes unintentional errors and still hold shared accountability when needed

- I listened with an open mind and did not cast judgments until I heard all sides.

- I gave honest but constructive feedback but made sure that my expectations were clear

- I intervened during difficult patient interactions.

- I did not condone workplace violence. I am an advocate for patient AND staff safety,

- I cried with the nurse, when she/he needed a shoulder to cry on.

- I am fair, tough but compassionate.

- I care. I only want the best for the unit, for the patients, and for the staff.

I am still learning…. My difference may not be as exciting and full of action as when I was in the front line, but I'm hoping that I make a difference to make the work experience easier for those in the trenches of providing care. I consider it a moral and ethical obligation to try my very best as a leader.

Part 2:
ED Covid-19 Nursing Diaries

This is not just my story. This is also a snapshot of my department's journey through the horrors of a pandemic, with all the heartaches and the small victories. Nobody comes out of this war unscathed.

It takes courage to go where nobody else wants to go.
It takes dedication to face this unfamiliar enemy.
It takes resilience to bounce back from a shift of heartaches to return the next day for more.
It takes sangfroid to be a health care worker at this time of great stress.
It takes someone special and amazing to be in the frontlines of this war.

We represent the healthcare workers in the middle of this fight against COVID-19.

SUPER HEROES

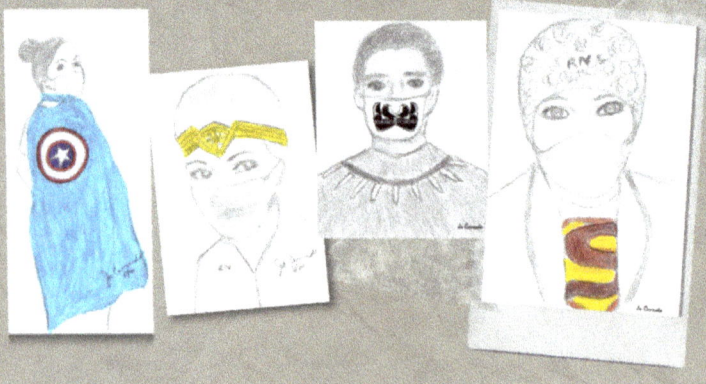

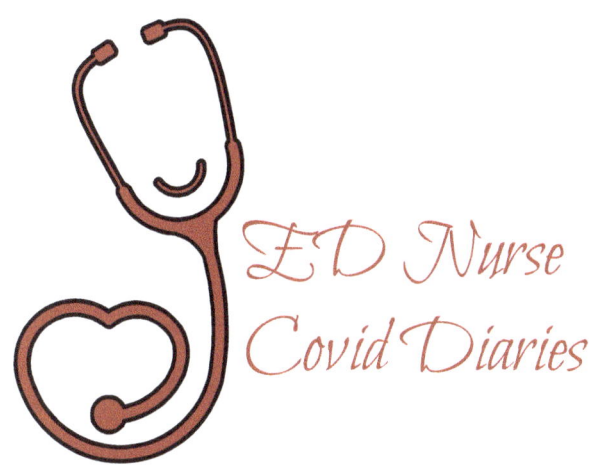

ED Nurse Covid Diaries

I believe in telling the stories of the frontline staff in the war against a scary disease. I want the world to understand our stories behind our masks and inside our hearts. I want to share our fears and hopes, our tears of sadness and joys, and our heartaches and the small victories.

Equipped with their personal protective equipment (PPE) of gowns, face shields, goggles, and N95 masks, the nurses, doctors, techs, and other ancillary staff ran towards the patients. Eerily reminiscent of how the firemen, the police, and EMS crews ran towards the World Trade Center buildings in 9/11.

The COVID-19 pandemic is a medical challenge beyond anyone's imagination. It is a puzzle of enormous complexity to all healthcare workers, all over the world. Our Emergency Department staff steps up to the plate to face an enemy they have not met before.

In this battle against the coronavirus, the warriors choose to give their utmost best amidst the anxiety, fear, and the stress. Strength, courage, and dedication defined our practice.

On these pages are the faces of the brave ones. Remember them.

It takes courage to go where nobody else wants to go.

It takes dedication to face this unfamiliar enemy.

It takes resilience to bounce back from a shift of heartaches to return the next day for more.

It takes sangfroid to be a health care worker at this time of great stress.

It takes someone special and amazing to be in the frontlines of this war.

We represent the healthcare workers in the middle of this fight against COVID-19.

January 1, 2020-

This will be a good year. This is the Year of the Nurse.

January 25-

China is far away; the danger of the coronavirus that devastated Wuhan is far away. (Or so, I thought). The hospital cautions us to prepare but there is a general sense that it's just like the FLU. The CDC says that the Flu killed more people than the Wuhan virus. I thought, we're safe here in America. Hey, even POTUS downplayed Wuhan. Life goes on.

February 17-

The Novel coronavirus is here. The DOH, CDC, and WHO issued their guidelines. At triage, get the travel history, check. Ask the patient if he has cough, fever, upper respiratory symptoms, check. If they're elderly, double-check. Mask yourself and mask the patient. Isolate. The Infection Control staff is overseeing our response. The algorithm was distributed to the staff. We got this.

February 28-

We received about three patients with fevers, cough, positive travel history and they were just mildly sick. It's not bad, I assured myself, I assured my staff. Who was I kidding? I am scared.

March 8-

What's going on? The hospital is full-on in Incident Command mode. There is a frenzy of activities; meetings after meetings in the Incident Command Center. It is like Central Command Headquarters where strategic plans are issued, where guidelines and protocols come from, where frantic requests for supplies, equipment, and personnel go, where tough decisions are to be made. The Senior Leadership has their hands full.

The projection was that we have about 3 weeks before the patients will use up the ventilators in the hospital. Three more weeks to get the extra staffing and extra supplies. We need more N95s. I am praying that we have more time to prepare.

In the ED, we continue with the "Don and doff" training. My head is spinning with things to do:

1. Write the standard work for Triage and Isolation of COVID PUIs.
2. Plan for Surge capacity, Look for alternate treatment areas.
3. Request more RN travelers and techs to help us out during the apex of the COVID patients
4. Request to redeploy former ED nurses back to the ED
5. Train procedural nurses to assist in the ED using Team Nursing.
6. Order more PPE supplies

Most importantly: Calm the masses.

March 11-

The World Health Organization has declared COVID-19 a pandemic. Now reaching global proportions affecting 114 countries. The news brought a frisson of fear down my spine. I texted my family in the Philippines and instructed them to stay at home, to shelter in place, to keep my 89 y/o mother safe. I called my son who lives two towns away from me. I made him promise that he will work from home, that he should never leave without a mask, that he should always wash his hands, He laughed at me indulgently and reminded me that he used to work in a research lab, and that he, of all people, knows how to thoroughly wash his hands. He knows he has to self-distance and to wear his mask every time he goes out. When we Face-timed, my son jokingly rolled his eyes at me then "virtually hugged" me. He knows I'm just being a mom.

March 12-

Fear. It is scary. Like going to the battlefield. We wonder, "Are we doing this right? Are we using the right PPE? Are we handwashing long enough?"

And yet we go to work. Every day. Despite our fears.

March 14-

My email to the nursing staff:

I know that there is not much we can say as we go through this COVID-19 crisis together. What I know is that the ED staff continues to give their very best despite the anxiety of the unknown. The emergency department itself can be chaotic and stressful. This is the nature of our work, and right now, your minds are probably spinning with the barrage of inservice, instructions, and simply the demands of being on the frontlines in this war. I just want to thank you for your amazing hard work and resilience. Thank you, thank you. If you have any questions, please do not hesitate to e-mail or call us (Anthony, Cynthia, Lauren, and I- even if you just want to vent). FYI, all the COVID-19 testing for our admitted PUI patients came back NEGATIVE, including the last one who went to the ICU (WR, 35 y/o male).

We are trying our very best to mitigate our current circumstances and to ease your workload during surges:

1. We are in the midst of finding alternate sites to move those who are Worried Well and those with mild symptoms than can be treated and released quickly. We will be using alternative areas to care for the surge of patients.

2. This week-end, we are piloting the use of the Ambulatory Care Clinic to refer the ESI 4-5 patients to decant the ED, thankfully with their own Ambulatory Care staff.

3. For admitted patients, more Isolation rooms were created in 7West and soon in 7E ICU for critical care surges.

What we ask of you is for you to be nice to each other. Watch each other's back and use the buddy system when you're donning and doffing. If you can come in for OT, please let us know, even if just to relieve for breaks. More than ever, we need you to come to work. And because we need to care for our own selves, try to Plan Your Joy. We're in this together.

March 15-

It's a Saturday spent at work. The ED is overcrowded with patients worried about their symptoms. We have the worried wells, but there are more patients coming with respiratory distress. We opened the ambulatory clinic on the second floor with the physician assistants and ambulatory clinic staff seeing those with mild-acuity symptoms.

This week, the ED leadership finalized our Surge plan and allocated other areas for COVID patients as we prepare for our projected Peak in two weeks. It is only Saturday and we're already in Phase 2, way ahead of schedule. Out of the 30 boarders in the ED, only two were not COVID. Today, we saw patients presenting with new symptoms and testing positive for COVID. It was a long, tiring day.

I ordered pizza for the staff. Doctors, nurses, and the ancillary staff all came running to the conference room. A nurse told me that she just needed a breather and just wanted to smell a good pepperoni pizza. I sat down to eat my ham and pineapple pizza pie, but did not have the strength to finish the whole thing. I had the feeling that things are going to get worse, then worst before it becomes better.

May God bless us all.

March 16-

Wow! A family with 4 kids from the community came to the ED to thank the staff for our service during this COVID-19 pandemic. They brought several pies of pizza with handwritten Thank You cards from the kids. The ED staff works hard every single day but has been totally amazing these past weeks amidst the fear and uncertainty. Being in the frontlines can be scary, but this gesture really warmed my heart. I am so glad that the staff is recognized for a job well done. I had my Joy late this afternoon after a full, exhausting day.

March 17-

I'm supposed to be off today but has been on the phone since 630am with back-to-back conference calls. Our hospital President just mentioned our ED with a special mention of my LinkedIn post about the community appreciation.

March 19-

We lost three patients in the ED today due to COVID. Their chest x-rays were horrible, "bilateral confluent diffuse airspace opacities". The doctors tried high flow oxygen, then BiPAP. But the patients were tiring out. They needed the ventilators to give them time to marshal their immunological response to the virus. It was frightening to witness the patients gasp for breath. It was gut-wrenching to be so helpless.

The ED was full, NEDOCs score was in the 160s with 40 boarders and five waiting for ICU beds. There was a sense of urgency as we tried to arrange for transfers to the floors. I made several calls to Admitting office. Where are the beds? I was frustrated but there was not much we can do until the beds open up upstairs. The Incident Command Center was directing the storm of activities to support the hospital operations and ensuring we have enough PPE. Although we are in scary times, I felt secure in the knowledge that the hospital leadership was truly responsive to our needs.

March 20-

I am the nursing director but I do not do direct bedside care like these brave men and women do. But I sure do my damn best to support them as best as I can do. I fight my own battles to secure more staff, more equipment, more supplies. I spend 10-12 hours in the hospital five days a week, and then we're expected to be on call for any emergencies. The nursing directors were just told that we have to do the Incident Management huddles at 830am even on Saturdays and Sundays. Even with all of these, it will certainly not compare with the higher risk that the bedside staff face every single day.

I received this text from a nurse: *"Today was a rough day with all the sick patients in the ED but having our EMS there was soooo helpful. They were so eager to step up and work. They were so interested in all the patients, treated them with so much respect and helped me out tremendously. If they weren't there, I think today easily could have been one of those days you go home and cry or bury your face in a pint of ice cream. I hope they come back every day and thank you for having them there."*

I felt feverish. My temperature was 97.8. Thank God.

March 22-

In the #YearoftheNurse2020, the COVID-19 pandemic is certainly challenging the resolve of nurses, and all the healthcare workers (doctors, PAs, techs, registrars, handlers, ancillary staff), all over the world. The Emergency Department staff steps up to the plate as they have done time and time again. In the war against this coronavirus, the warriors choose to give their best amid the anxiety, fear, and the stress. Strength, courage, and dedication are manifested in every single one of them, no matter what their job entails. These are the faces of the brave ones, those who uphold their duty above all else. Thank you everyone, as well as the other warriors in the inpatient units and in the ICUs. I am so proud of all of the healthcare workers here and everywhere.

As you can see, the community acknowledges all our efforts. The food just keeps on coming, a gesture of appreciation from the people who depend on us for their healthcare needs. The Thank Yous certainly mean a lot; they remind us of the reason why we are doing this. We are working for the patients who need our care. This is one department's journey in pictures, chronicles of individual and the ED team strengths. I started my COVID-19 album on Facebook. I wanted to capture in posterity those moments of levity in between moments of heartbreaks. We will survive this madness.

March 24-

The nerves were getting to the staff. As the handlers were giving out the new goggles, there was a misunderstanding about the distribution. I got to the ED right when one nurse burst into tears, she was frustrated because she did not get her new goggles, and she was holding her flimsy old ones with the frayed strings. I mediated and got her the new goggles that she deserved. I know that the tears were of frustration, were of fear. I could only pat her back and stay by her side until her tears stopped. She did not want to leave her assignment. Then she took a deep breath and smiled, "I am okay."

The RN travelers are not here yet, but at least some Procedural nurses and techs were redeployed back to the ED. They can do tasks, labs and lines, Team Nursing we go. Then, we received some EMS techs and paramedics arrived. All hands on deck. We needed all the assistance we can get. The doctors and nurses have been rushing to the rooms to resuscitate the sick patients who come right after another. I saw one of the doctors sitting at the desk with anguish on his face. He just called the patient's son that his father passed away. The apex came two weeks early.

March 25-

The nurse manager and educator were out on furlough, half of my leadership team. My assistant nurse manager was busy trying to staff the unit. For the first time in all my years as an ED nurse, I felt I was drowning. The ED NEDOCs score was high in the 170s, we are seriously overcrowded with two intubations going at the same time. I kept an eye on the ventilator reports. We are low on the BiPAP but we're getting some delivered in the afternoon. The hospital converted some inpatient units to ICU beds but our patients were not going up quick enough to decant the ED. I must say that I am impressed on how the hospital converted some units into COVID-receiving units in a matter of days.

APEX. The apex came two weeks early. A 55- year-old COVID patient succumbed to cardiac arrest. Too young to die. It could be anyone of us. There was shock in the nurses' eyes. After he was pronounced dead, the team members offered a moment of silence to pay their respects to the patient. There was no family to mourn him at the bedside. We made sure that none of our patients died alone.

HELPLESSNESS. I tried to help out with the post-mortem but the nurses told me that they can handle it. One nurse said, "We cannot afford you to be sick. Who else will look out for us?" I almost bawled in front of the team. I felt a little bit useless and yet somewhat useful, even needed. I realized that we both have our tasks to do in this war against the pandemic.

March 26-

My nurse's husband was admitted to the hospital for shortness of breath related to COVID-19 and she could not stay with him. No visiting rule, even for her. It broke her heart to be so helpless. I cannot do anything. As she cried on the phone, all I could do was listen and cry along with her. I called the nurse manager in that inpatient unit to keep an eye on the husband. I visited the unit but the patient was asleep. His breathing was normal and his oxygen saturation was 96% on nasal cannula. He will be okay. At least, my nurse's husband is not in the ICU.

I heard two medical codes being called in the ICUs in just one hour. There were more calls for the respiratory therapists throughout the day. The ED is like a warzone, we are a COVID unit after all. I saw a blur of yellow isolation gowns when a group of doctors and nurses responded to Room 22 in the ED; they have to intubate the new patient. Not even five minutes later, another call of help in Room 1 for a high flow oxygen machine. And another patient in respiratory distress was rushed in by EMS. The charge nurse called out for another team to Room 2. I had 36 boarders in the ED, all complaints related with COVID, some confirmed, some PUIs, some PUMs. The nomenclatures and the changing guidelines from CDC are confusing. The intensity level is high in the ED.

March 27-

Suddenly, there were videos of clapping and cheering emanating from the apartment buildings around Manhattan; New Yorkers rallying to support those who cannot stay home. They were united in celebrating the healthcare professionals working in the front lines of the COVID-19 pandemic. It felt good. This is our "WHY".

March 28-

After an exhausting week of being the Administrator on Call in the middle of a brutal week of COVID-19 response in the hospital, I needed to do self-care in order to get re-energized for probably a more brutal week. And then reading the Thank You cards from the community, I see the reason "Why" we are doing this. This is our "Ikigai", our reason for being. The ED received an outpouring of love and support from the community. Food deliveries came unsolicited almost every day. And they were calling the healthcare workers their heroes.

Late at night, I received a call from my assistant nurse manager about the Visiting rules. A family member wanted to see her dying mother in the ED. The No Visitor rule was just enforced, but for end-of-life moments, visiting was allowed. The iPADs help with facilitating communication between families but nothing can take the place of an actual visit. The unit leaders all said yes. My chief nursing officer and chief medical officer approved. It was a humane decision to allow a daughter to say her final goodbye. No one should die alone.

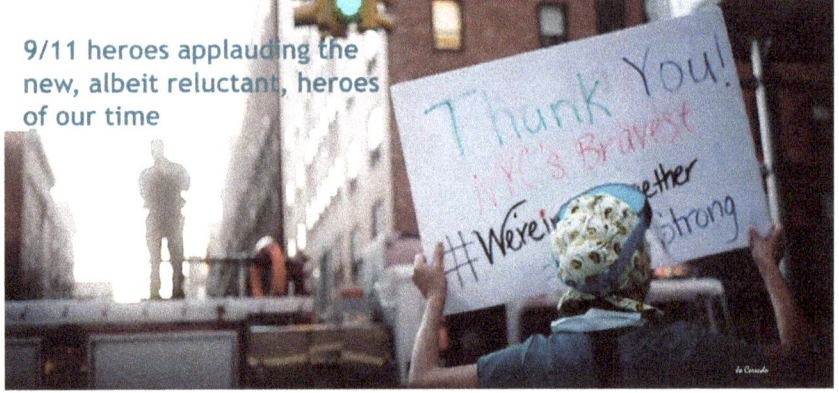

9/11 heroes applauding the new, albeit reluctant, heroes of our time

April 1-

The firemen from across the street were outside our ER with their huge fire trucks. NYPD joined in their clapping amid the Thank You's from people in the community. It was surreal.

A wall of heroes applauding the new, albeit reluctant, heroes of our time. The ED staff loved returning the applause. The rousing celebration of the work we do somehow validates all the sacrifices that we make. There were air horns and sirens, somewhere distant the clanging of pots and pans. Soon the ED staff was joined by other hospital workers from the inpatient units.

The ED staff hooted and cheered, for a few minutes forgetting the horrors behind the front door of the ED. In moments of crisis, we savor those moments which makes sense of everything we do.

April 3-

As I go through the ED, I see all the staff bravely going through the day. I had to peer into their face shields to see who I was talking to. Wearing their masks and face shields, they put their thumbs up but I could feel the rising anxiety.

The eyes told me what they were feeling. SAD eyes from the deaths they have witnessed, more than they ever did in a single shift. WORRIED eyes because they needed assurance that they will not bring this virus home to their family. HAUNTED eyes for witnessing the final goodbyes between the patients and their loved ones on the iPAD.

In the staff lounge, on her break, a nurse removed her tight N95 mask as she settled down on a chair to rest, the string marks stayed on her face; red bruises under her eyes and on her nose. She replaced her N95 with a surgical mask. She closed her eyes, probably in meditation, probably just to get her bearing. Like everyone else in the healthcare world, she was exhausted. I closed the door so she can have her moment of peace.

But they are here, doing their job the best that they could. It's the worst of times but I see the staff stepping up. A physician assistant brought an iPAD to the room so the patient and the self-quarantined family can talk to each other. The doctors slumped on their seats as they held their phones to their ears, as they fielded questions from the worried families. The nurses and techs gowned up to prepare a patient to the morgue. At 3pm, the techs gathered around after huddle to say their prayers. They are the heroes of these uncertain times. And to survive, I see them supporting and being kind to each other, sharing the hand-made masks and surgical caps donated to them by worried friends.

April 6-

The hospital released the video that the Marketing Department made, of the staff dancing; taking a respite from the heartbreaking work to just enjoy ourselves and to support each other through the hard times. Somehow, we found time to just have a little fun, and at the same time exhort the public to stay home. #stayhome #flattenthecurve

https://www.youtube.com/watch?v=qZ3C2AESRmQ&t=12s

April 7-

Positive news of survival should be celebrated. In our fight against COVID, we have to gather strength and hope in those things that affirm our impact on our patients' lives. We have to find the joys that will keep us moving forward. The digital board in the lobby announced that there were 137 patients who went back home to their loved ones yesterday. Today, my nurse's husband was number 138. Finding our Joy in small victories.

A staff nurse who was out on sick leave called me crying. She saw the staff video and expressed her guilt for not taking her place at the bedside with her peers. Other staff members expressed the same thing to me. I told her gently to take care of herself first, that the best thing she can do for us is to just keep us in her prayers.

A week ago, I suggested to the Incident Command Center to post the Good News of our discharges, as kind of a morale-booster to the staff, to remind them that we are saving lives.

These are our finest hours indeed. I wondered if our city will give the healthcare workers our own ticker tape parade, maybe in the Canyon of Heroes. I hope soon.

April 8-

This never gets old. A much-needed boost from our friends at FDNY, heroes themselves. There are new chalkmarks of appreciation on the sidewalks leading to the ED, all from the community, their own little way of appreciating the hospital staff. This time, the firemen were joined by the NYPD officers on horses. I saw my nurses' eyes filled with tears of joy and gratitude.

April 10-

PAUSE AND APPLAUSE.

We PAUSE to reflect on the lives lost due to COVID-19 and to strengthen our resolve to fight for the lives we can still save.

APPLAUSE is a more joyous occasion. We clap when a patient is discharged. We dance when the music "Call on Me' plays. We applaud to rejoice for the life that was saved; someone's loved one who was given a second chance.

I am glad I was able to witness a patient's discharge; he is a COVID survivor. The patient broke into a wide grin as he was met with a chorus of well-wishes and boisterous applause at the hospital lobby. It is an honor and privilege to be among a group of people who cheered this patient. Much as he appreciated the warm send-off, I felt as similarly blessed. It was a great feeling, a much-needed pick-me-up. There was encouraging news about the downward trending admission rates but I couldn't shake a lingering sadness earlier because of some losses of people I know.

At that moment, I was energized. I caught his eyes and I felt my own tears fall as he said, "Thank You". I never took care of him, but he was everybody's patient at that time.

I felt joyful seeing the patient's smiling eyes above his mask. I needed that. "Sir, Thank you."

April 12-

"Always call upon our Father
When afflictions, you may suffer;
He'll never forsake you in your hardship.
His help He will give as long as you shall live"

This I believe. I had to believe that the pandemic will soon end. Our worship service is now on Webex. The video was grainy, the choir hymns were canned, but the minister delivered a spiritual and uplifting sermon. My church (Church of Christ) has been doing the virtual worship service by Webex for several weeks now. I miss going to Church; I miss the brethren, the hymn-singing, just being in the House of God. This is just a bump in the road, a little test of faith. After the service, the minister beamed with relief when he saw the faces on the screen. We waved back at him. My soul needed it.

April 13-

One of the nurses relayed that she triaged one of the first COVID 19 patients she took care of last month. She recognized the eyes of the patient; those same eyes who looked at her with dread when he came in with double pneumonia and had to be intubated on his first visit. She thought he was the sickest of the sickest that horrendous day with a poor prognosis. But he was discharged two weeks later. This time he came because he was short of breath on exertion.

As he sat on the triage chair, he relaxed and even laughed when the nurse stated she recognized him. His eyes were not as frightened anymore, just concerned. He later smiled with relief when his oxygen saturation showed as 99% on room air. He acknowledged he just had to give time to feel stronger, for his lungs to go back to normal. Nurse Jovy told me that she sobbed in relief when the patient left to go home.

April 14-

After a heart-breaking loss of a church friend that had

momentarily shook my world, one particular patient discharge somehow eases the pain, even for just a little moment.

One of our own ED staff, a registrar, was discharged after weeks of hospitalization for COVID-19. The word Social Distancing did not really enter my consciousness at that time, sorry. In defense, everyone was all masked.

The lobby of the hospital was filled with thundering applause amid chants of his name. It was a celebration of a life saved, of winning one against a dreaded disease, of teamwork and unity, of survival (not just for the patient but for all those who continue to fight).

Joining this celebration was one of my nurses who survived COVID herself. She was one of the loudest cheerers. Seeing both survivors was inspiring. The moment was all-powerful, and a big morale-booster for those in the biggest battle in our professional lives. It was a joyful celebration of the men and women who fought for this patient. As I saw the numbers on the Discharge monitor continue to climb, I am hopeful that this nightmare will soon pass. It was a special Thank You that another one got away. Take that, COVID!!!

April 15-

SADNESS IN MY HEART. I feel a deep, aching sadness in my heart. Yesterday, one of the most-beloved members of our church passed away. I cried for the family he left behind and for the generations of church brethren that he touched. I cried for every single one of my friends and acquaintances who died due to COVID. There is a pain of loss and the continuing fear of losing some more. Too many friends who lost family members to this pestilence. Too many precious lives gone.

And then I listened as they shared their fears. I could only listen. And sometimes I cried with them

April 16-

There are others in other states with a myopic understanding of how dangerous this coronavirus is and they demand to ease the lockdown. The healthcare workers continue to venture out everyday to take care of the sick so that others can stay home. I feel anger that there are people who bemoan about being bored out of their minds due to staying at home. I feel disgust at those who disregard the tragedy of lives lost just because they think that their freedom is curtailed.

The Stop-the-lockdown movement is fueled by ignorant, uneducated people who were not yet touched by this pandemic. They are just adult versions of that stupid teenager during the spring break in Miami who stated, "If I get corona, I get corona. At the end of the day, I'm not going to let it stop me from partying.".

What is wrong with these people?

April 20-

I must have looked dejected as I walked through the lobby. I had my surgical cap and my N95 mask on but I was still recognizable with my ubiquitous white lab coat. Somebody asked me "How are you?". I shrugged my shoulders, squeaked a weak "I'm okay", and quickly turned around.

My tears threatened to overwhelm me and I did not want to ugly-cry in the middle of the lobby. A part of me wanted to say "I'm having a tough time" but I was not ready to share. In my previous hospital, five hospital workers succumbed to the complications of Covid-19. I worry about my friends and family. I do not want to lose any more friends to this disease. Some of my nurses are still on furlough. The threat of contamination looms over our heads like Damocles' sword.

I managed to get to my office and pulled the tight mask off my face. I closed the door and cried my heart out.

April 23-

This morning looks like a miracle to me. I can breathe better. I had a good night sleep after the surprisingly calming effects of my crossword puzzles and the soothing music of Anne Murray. Earlier that day, the Mental Health Liaison met with the staff to offer some options to de-stress, to decompress. We need to do our Mental PPE. I prayed not for myself but for my own family and my work family. Then, I turned to the one thing that always calms me down: I write. I wrote what my heart spoke.

There were only 8 patients in the ED, three of which are COVID patients waiting for the med-surg beds. No ICU patient at this time. More nurses than there were patients. For the very first time ever, our NEDOCS score is -2 (negative 2). The charge nurse later texted me in the afternoon that the volume had picked up. There were now 40 patients in the ED with some trauma codes and non-COVID patients in the mix.

Face-Time eased my loneliness when I spoke with my son. He had just been working at home and he is safe. My mom is also safe in Manila, enjoying her wine now that there was no more beer to procure. It is how she relaxes at home. Everybody at home and at work are safe. That's all I needed to know.

My temperature was 97.8F. Most of my staff members who were furloughed are back to work, ready to join the fight again. Governor Andrew Cuomo said that the COVID-19 war is not over but he cautions against prematurely stopping the lockdown.

The tsunami of admissions had abated. Yes, it's not over yet, but there is light at the end of the tunnel.

May 10-

I am just amazed that despite the constraints of the COVID crisis, we are still able to be creative with our Nurses Week celebrations. We even did Dancing in the Street. It is the Year of the Nurse. We will survive.

June 12-

Nine minutes. It took nine minutes to kill a man. George Floyd's death is so much shocking with its brutality and an unconscionable disregard for life.

Today, June 2nd, the hospital staff stood in solidarity with our Black brothers and sisters. We joined our fellow humans in a peaceful protest for a person to be given the same right and privilege to live on this earth. We filled the street in front of the hospital, all colors standing together in solidarity. As we worked side by side with each other during the pandemic, we join our hands to fight racism. I am proud of the solidarity we showed. We raised the banner "Enough is Enough". Then we paused for remembrance. That was the longest nine minutes ever.

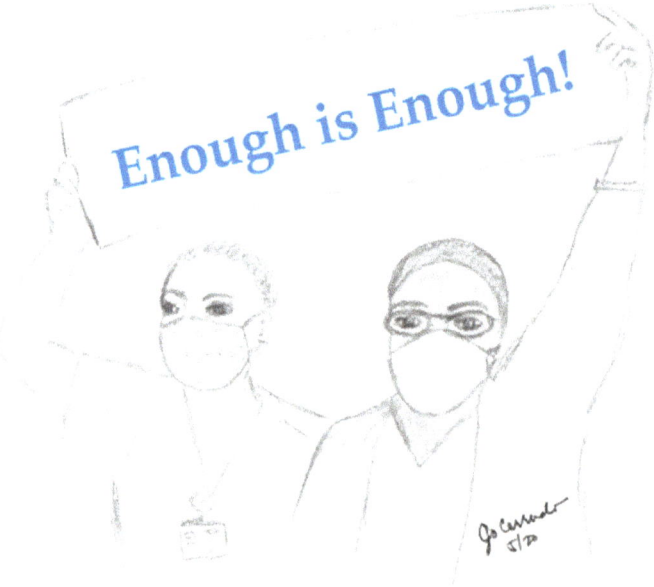

July 30-

What a year it is. It's not over yet. The tsunami of admissions had abated here in New York but there is still fear of a second wave. There are more non-COVID patients in the ED. The patient census had dramatically gone down. There are more nurses than patients. Now I can breathe better. I am sleeping better. There is light at the end of the tunnel.

Sept. 29, 2020-

To heal myself, I turn to the things that I am grateful for: my family and friends, my church, my work family, music, books, food, puzzles, and our dog. I look for my joy-triggers. That is how I keep myself sane amidst all the challenges of life in the new-normal. For self-care, I continue with my Covid Diary. I write so I can continue to be strong, for me, my family, and my staff.

October 4-

I hear laughter now.

I see my staff SMIZE; their eyes are smiling above their masks. They know it is not completely over yet, but they find strength in each other.

Nobody comes out of this pandemic unscathed. We have to actively and deliberately plan our joys in and outside of work.

As we all put together the pieces of our broken hearts, we march onward, stronger together.

December 13-

The second wave is here. Covid 2.0. It is a scary time. But the vaccine is here. There is HOPE and RELIEF. It is the beginning of the end. I am hoping that a few months from now, I can finally travel and hug my mom again.

For us. For our families. For you. For our country.

December 17-

I got my Covid-19 vaccine today and so did some of my ED and ICU colleagues. Finally, the Pfizer vaccine is here. I have been waiting for this. Now that we're on the Second Wave of this horrific pandemic, I am confident that we have what it takes to fight back with a vengeance. I am joyful that this is the beginning of the end of this disease that has gripped us in a chokehold for so many months.

The healthcare workers went through a heart-wrenching period, of personal losses, of profound sadness, of fears and anxieties that continue to haunt us to this day.

But now there is hope. I must confess that I was teary-eyed because I can see the light at the end of the long tunnel. The vaccine is a game-changer. This will afford all of mankind to get back to new-normal. Thank you to the scientists and the volunteer research subjects; they are heroes themselves.

#LetsBeatCOVID19 #Havefaithinthescience

December 31-

It was a heart-wrenching year. A year of profound sadness, of despair and helplessness, of fears and anxieties that continue to haunt us to this day. This disease has gripped us in a chokehold for so many months.

Somehow, the collection of pictures turned into a journal of our collective experience during the pandemic. I encouraged others to share their personal reflections; I understand the need to share, to relieve the heart of the burden of fear.

The ED staff fought together, united as we were never before. We had to work together as a team; it was the only way to survive in these darkest of days.

For me, Journaling is a coping mechanism, it puts things in perspective; it slows things down to manageable parts. It is a therapeutic activity to drain the brain of stressful recollections. It gives me time to breathe, to process my emotions.

When written on paper, the pain loses its intensity. Like a catharsis of the negative emotions. Not that we can ever forget. We just need to keep our hearts from breaking into a million pieces, just need to find comfort in the small triumphs. Just so we can continue to fight and survive.

The war against Covid-19 is ongoing, but having the vaccine is a huge relief. We have a fighting chance.

As 2020 closes... HOPE. Looking forward to 2021 be a better and safer year for all of us.

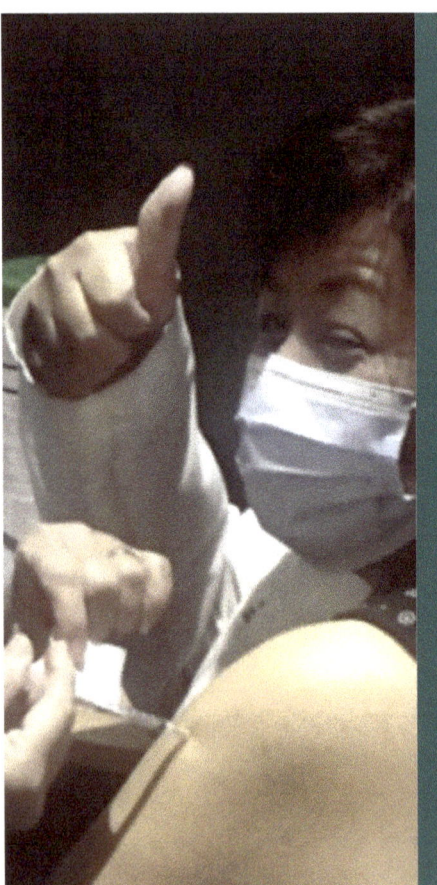

HAPPINESS IS...

*Getting the Covid-19 vaccine.
Seeing the light at the end of the tunnel.
Hoping for the near-normal.
Dreaming of traveling and hugging my mom again.*

LET'S DO IT!

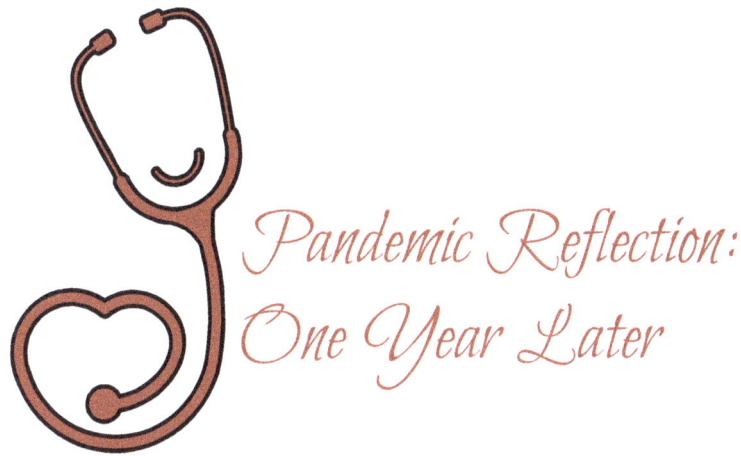

Pandemic Reflection: One Year Later

March 11, 2021-

Today is a moment of reflection for all of us. Last year on March 11, the World Health Organization declared COVID-19 a global pandemic. I wrote this in my journal, not knowing that Covid will still persist as a menace a year later. The loss of lives is still staggering and so emotional. Two more losses, one was an agency companion/sitter at work and another a church member in the prime of her life. When will this pandemic end? I did not expect to hear of sad news so close to home, when we're almost on the homestretch.

Today, we gathered in the Resus Room to pay respects and remember our co-worker. Although she was not a full-time hospital employee, we claimed her as our own because she was assigned to the ED from her agency for 4 years. JT was an agency employee sent to watch patients who were emotionally disturbed, suicidal, or patients who are Fall and elopement risks. It was not an easy job; the patients were challenging, but she persevered and tried to help as much as they could, when she was sometimes sick herself.

The room was filled with nurses, techs, and other ancillary workers. It started slow but soon the staff was sharing their memories of her. The chaplain led us in prayer. It was difficult to hold back the tears because I did not think that one year later, we will still be mourning the deaths of people we know. I didn't know that I needed the hug. The staff had a good cry then we dried our tears as we went back to work.

This second wave of Covid was not as intense as the first wave, but what is unrelenting is the slow road to recovery. Maybe it is our impatience to return back to normal. Maybe it's the frustration that people still die, despite all the things we have learned.

One year later, my son is still safe and we have been indulging in our food trips, mask and all. My 90 y/o mom is socially-distancing in our home, with all her needs catered to by my family. We did her birthday celebration via Zoom on February 14th. And I had my vaccine.

In reflection, I realized that coming out of this terrible period is doable. There is light at the end of this tunnel. We have to take care of ourselves, still seek those things that give joy to our lives, hold on for those moments of triumph, celebrate the lives we have saved, give thanks for the science of the vaccine, and rejoice for the grace and blessings of having survived through it all. Simply put, just keep on hanging in there. I look forward to the future of hope.

Part 3:
In the Future

Looking forward to what lies ahead

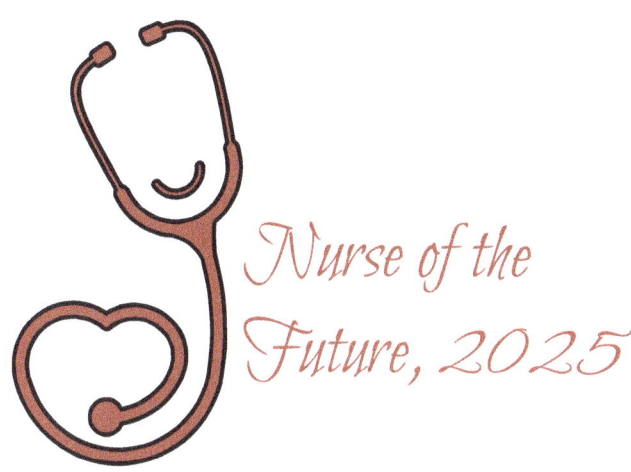

Nurse of the Future, 2025

SEPTEMBER 2025

It's time to say goodbye to her 'virtual' nursing cap. Dr. Jade Marciano is ready to hang up her stethoscope, finally. After all, she had been working as a nurse for 42 years now. After completing her Doctorate of Nursing Practice degree 10 years ago, she had moved on to the executive leadership position in the hospital.

"Hi, Tita Jade. I will miss your daily stops." Her niece Charlene gave her a quick buzz on the cheek before she ran over to the ambulance ramp to meet the EMS trauma notification. Charlene is the senior nurse practitioner on duty.

Nurse practitioners had finally been integrated into the fabric of ED care. It had taken years of resistance from the medical community, but after the exorbitant malpractice insurance costs had driven down enrollment in medical schools, the emergency attending physicians had begrudgingly accepted the NPs to practice alongside the EM residents.

Dr. Jade chuckled at the thought of one clueless senatorial what's-her-name candidate who had tried to belittle the nurses in her native country by implying that the student nurses could get by with limited education. Her concept of "room nurses" had angered the Filipino nurses, and she eventually lost the election in 2013. In her wildest imagination, she probably did not even think that nurses would even rise in stature even more.

The 2010 Institute of Medicine's landmark report had been quite a revelation in its success. The hospital had achieved an unprecedented 100% BSN-prepared nursing staff, belying the prediction of a nursing shortage by 2020. A remarkable 35% of the ED RNs has Masters' degree, and had been utilized as Senior Staff Nurses 5th level, with expanded responsibilities as patient care navigators and evidence-based practice advocates. The ED administration had wisely adjusted their staff by providing more Patient Care Techs and other ancillary staff to offset the higher salaries of these advanced practice RNs.

Dr. Jade is a prime example of the IOM's vision. She was trailblazer in her profession, having collaborated with the physicians to introduce new care initiatives. She agreed that the public's and medical community's perception of nurses had greatly been turned around when faced with more educated nurses.

"Trauma Team, Resus 51", a melodic announcement interrupted Dr. Jade's thoughts. A patient from a multi-vehicular accident had just been wheeled by EMS, with a mechanical compressor performing CPR on the bloodied patient. There was no time for an intubation in the field.

In the age of microchips, only the most privacy-concerned patient would have an unknown medical history. The triage nurse bar-scanned the patient's wrist and soon the patient's recent medical history was displayed on a medical I-Pad Patient Screen under the cardiac monitor. The patient was an open book, a reality (and a necessity) in Big Brother's world.

Mr. C was a 35 year-old man with an AICD from a cocaineinduced cardiomyopathy. The EM-NP quickly deactivated the AICD. A glove EKG remained on the patient's torso, a far cry from the bulb-suction EKG electrodes of Dr. Jade's student years.

The ED attending wrapped a DBAC (Deep Bleeder Acoustic Coagulation) cuff on the patient's upper arm to seal an arterial bleed. The trauma surgeon then activated the ultrasound zap to coagulate the severed vessel. The nurse had started her Trauma Bleed cocktail- Tranexamic acid (antifibrinolytic), Kefpush (an IV push antibiotic), and Tetanus toxoid.

The EM-NP also had started an intraosseus line and gave a Blood Substitute polyheme on the accident scene; a necessary intervention in a depleted Blood Bank supply. There was no need for cross-matching; no chance for a transfusion reaction.

The ED attending stopped the compressor to check for the pulse. The patient pulse was steady and bounding, Sinus tachycardia was reflected on a sleek touch screen. The patient was still unconscious and was having labored breathing.

"BP 90/62, HR-120, O2 sat 92% on 100% non-rebreather.", the nurse announced just loud enough to be heard by the Trauma Team, as well as to record the vitals on the lapel mike that was attached to her Dragoneer Head set. The hands-free device allows her to tape her assessments while she assists with patient care. As soon as she would have the time, she would review then accept the recordings on her own hospital-issued mobile phone to be written into the permanent electronic chart. Most of the nurses preferred the mike than typing into their mobile device.

NP Charlene assisted the Trauma resident in intubation and administered the dosage-controlled bar-coded RSI meds via the brachial line, and soon the resident inserted a Glidescope for easy tracheal intubation.

"ETT to vent, Tidal volume 500, F1O2 100%, AC rate 0f 16". The trauma nurse continued to intone into her mike, as the respiratory therapist connected the endotracheal tube to the new compact-sized three-pound portable ventilator.

The trauma nurse had sent the blood tubes on the Chute to Lab, but gave the smaller sample tube to the Patient Care Tech for bedside testing.

The Patient Care Tech keyed in the results of point-of-care hematocrit, lactate and basic metabolic panel and transmitted the results on the Patient Screen. The ED attending reviewed the trended results, and nodded with satisfaction on the improved hematocrit level.

The Trauma attending brought out his newest gadget to show off, a hand-held body ultrasound scanner to check on a possible aortic dissection or any vaso-aneurysm. There was none, and suppressing a disappointed sigh, he called for the x-ray technician to come into the room.

The technician turned on the switch and the portable multi-purpose x-ray/MRI scanner lowered down from the ceiling. A series of clicks and lights emanated from the machine, creating a surreal glow around the patient.

A lacerated liver was displayed on the Patient Screen. Snapping to attention, a gaggle of trauma residents started to disconnect the patient from the cardiac monitor.

Even with the sophisticated and ultra-modern technology, the doctors still did not know how to calmly prepare the patient for transport, without unhooking the wrong tubes and tangling the IV lines. In their haste, they just wasted precious time. The nurses quickly took over, and finally declared the patient ready to go.

It all happened in twenty minutes, and off to the OR did the patient go. The RFID tracker recorded the patient's move.

An audible decrease in the decibel and excitement level in the ED coincided with the patient's transfer. And soon, the ED was back to its usual non-trauma frenetic pace.

Dr. Jade surveyed the newly-renovated ED, and decided that she will again propose more beds to be added. The patient daily census still remained in the 500s because of more hospital closings. The medical scene would remain a challenge.

Back at her corner Penthouse office, Dr. Jade enjoyed a 180-view of Brooklyn and Manhattan. It is a good feeling to have gone through it all. She had emerged triumphant.

From a simple nursing student in the Philippines in the late 70's, where the students used to help sterilize the glass syringes and needles, make their own cotton balls, reuse most supplies, and carry the metal patient charts for the doctors with their superior airs.

When she moved to the United States in the early 1980's, she was thrust into a chronic care hospital. With 40 patients under her care, she was introduced to functional nursing. Most times, she gave out meds with only a 2x2 index card with transcribed hand-written medication orders.

In the 1990's, she entered the world of emergency nursing and she was hooked. It was a world in transition. The nurses had to prove themselves against some medical doctors who could not believe that nurses should have a voice.

The 2000s was a year for innovations, and medical breakthroughs. Electronic charting decreased medical errors. And nursing was poised to take bigger roles in hospital leadership. In 2012, she started her Simulation journey. Now, all her nurses prepare for real-life nursing with mandatory intensive simulation experience in the state-of-the-art Sim Lab.

Now, in 2025, the transformed nursing workforce had fulfilled its promise to take a much-deserved equal acknowledgement from the public. Somehow, the world had embraced the new and expanded roles of the nurse. An empowered nurse.

Yes, it's time to retire.

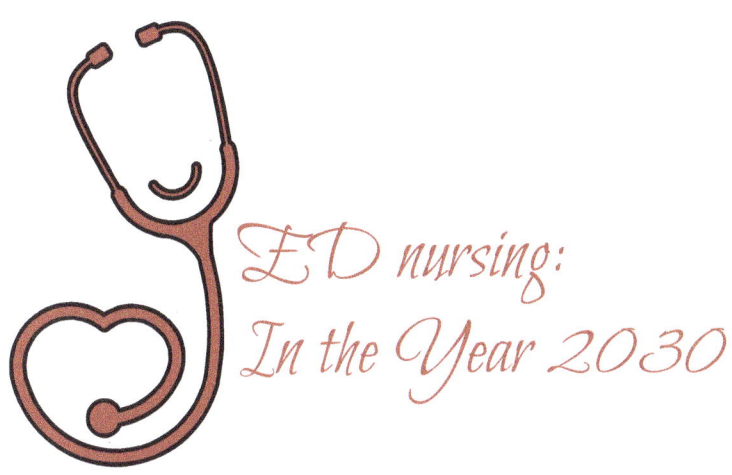

ED nursing: In the Year 2030

January 8, 2030- Into the Future

Nurse Jess entered the Emergency Department with her trademark walk, hopping with every other step, swinging her arms as she went straight to the Charge Nurse Station. As the Director of Nursing, she could have just looked at the dashboard on her Mango watch/minicomputer/phone to see the unit metrics. But she likes being in the middle of the action. Besides, her usually unflappable charge nurse Mae seemed a little bit frazzled as she answered her Comdevice, and mumbled something about "Remember 2020".

Jess entered the ED where she had been a nurse for 20 years, the last two years as the much-respected nursing director. Finally, they are in the new ED wing, a state-of-the art facility. Thanks to the generosity of the family of a prominent New York trillionaire. The 78-year-old man came in with a broken femur after a nasty fall, but was so impressed by the efficiency of the ED staff before he was whisked to the OR. He lingered on just in time to say his goodbyes to his family, but he made them promise to build a new ER. And the family donated billions of dollars to create an ED well-suited to meet the demands of a new Covid19-like crisis. No more hallway patients, every patient in their own private room with some amenities like a tv, electronic patient tracker, and a nurse-call device.

Jess outfitted in the hospital-mandated IRC (Infection Repellent Clothing) for this new disease outbreak from Texas. The Tyvek 3rd edition suit is very light with its own breathing apparatus the size of her hand. Her face shield mask is clear and does not fog nor suffocate. The plastic material covers her entire face and connects to the Tyvek suit itself. Thankfully, this new disease is not anywhere as virulent and as overwhelming as COVID-19. A shudder went through Jess' body as she remembered the year 2020, the Year of the Nurse which nobody ever anticipated to turn out to be a nightmare year for every healthcare worker. In the year 2030, it looks like they're in a repeat of 2020.

Last month, ten years ago was a distant memory, relegated to the hospital archives. Right after the nth ZoomstatCom meeting with the Infection Control Czar last week, the hospital leadership went into UltraPreparedness/Response Mode. The Incident Commander declared in his authoritative voice, "We are now in ICS level 2 and we expect to be in Level 3 soon."

After the meeting, she scrolled back on her personal online blog to look for her Covid Diaries. In 2020, the ED was declared an endemic area. Ground Zero or more accurately, the war zone, for the hospital as the patients came in gasping for breath and the ED staff rushed in to fight for the patients to survive. The staff heroically stepped up to the plate, buried their emotions, and proceeded to take care of the patients. It was a whole year unlike any other that no one in his right mind would ever want to go back to. In one of the Covid-19 memes, The "Back to the Future's" Emmett Brown admonished Marty McFly not to ever go to 2020 with his time travel machine.

Jess did not have to peruse the blog to relive the memories. Her heart ached in remembrance. She thinks she had some form of PTSD from that event, just like some of her colleagues. Thankfully, she was able to draw strength from her family and friends, as well as from her ED work family. Going through Covid hell proved how resilient healthcare workers are.

"Thank God, you're here!", Mae uttered in relief. She was still in nursing school when Covid-19 exploded. She heard terror stories from all the senior nurses, but now, her wild-eyed look resembled what Jess' 2020 nurses looked like. There was still several of those bad-ass nurses around; their eyes are calmer now, their experience during the Covid war gave them steel of nerves, and today, they serve as inspiration to their younger colleagues.

Jess swallowed her fear and made sure her smile reached her eyes above her mask. As the nursing director, she had to be a tower of strength, a source of truth, a comforting presence, and a purveyor of hope. Even if she felt a little apprehension as she saw the electronic dashboard in the Nurses station with the throughput metrics and unit statuses highlighted in Red. It has not changed through the years, we still use the Red Surge as common language that the ED is in crisis.

Dr. Johnson sauntered to the Nurses' station. Like Jess, Brad experienced Covid-19. He wore his veteran status with honor, which in a way, comforted his fellow doctors. Jess and Brad are ten years older now, wiser and toughened by their experience. Jess consulted with Brad and they decided to call a unit huddle.

Mae's voice crackled over the staff's Communication devices that were clipped on their scrubs. Except for those currently involved in a patient's care, most of the unit staff gathered in the 5-bedded Resuscitation room. Unable to maintain physical distancing, the nurses, doctors, techs, pharmacists, registrars, environmental services members, transporters, respiratory therapists, case managers, and even the paramedics attended the huddle.

Brad addressed the whole staff, "Ladies and gentlemen, we are at this point of declaring the ED as an endemic unit. Meaning, you will have to be in full PPE when you enter the ED door. Don't give me this crap that you cannot breathe because our masks are hundred times more comfortable than we have in 2020. We cannot afford to have some of you out sick. Use your PPE".

Jess addressed the staff. Knowing that everyone is compliant with the Covid and flu vaccine, she proceeded to tell the staff that another similar mRNA vaccine is being tested by the scientists. There will be some protection from the Covid vaccine, but this new vaccine will be specifically targeting this new disease called Joslin30.

Jess reviewed the surge and escalation protocol. Although the

NEDOCs score is high, all the patients are secured in their private rooms, most of which are with negative pressures. The patients have their own sophisticated TeleFam monitors to connect with their families remotely. Visiting hours was suspended except for special circumstances. The newly-reorganized CDC Fauci organization issued a much-vetted Joslin30 treatment algorithm which is immediately started in the ED. The point-of-care Joslin30 screening test is top-of-the-line accurate with a one-minute result time. Additional medical and nursing staff reinforcement from the National Medical Guard will be in the ED in two days. Supplies and equipment, and most importantly the ventilators are well-stocked. Three additional hospital units are being prepared for additional patients and will be available in a few hours.

As Jess relayed all the updates, she could see the staff visibly breathing in relief. They needed to hear that the updates; needed to hear that no patients have died so far, that patients are responding to the aggressive drug cocktail. Jess herself believed that the world is much-better prepared for this new challenge. They clapped at the end of Jess' summary of the ED status. She brought them hope and confidence that this crisis will soon pass.

"This is 2030, not a repeat of 2020. This time, we have an intelligent and responsible President who does not quarrel with her own Infection Control chief. This time, the science we trusted in 2020 is bringing us a new vaccine soon. This time, the government officials are on the same page. This time, our hospital is prepared for all eventualities. This time, we will get through this in just a month or so. Thank God, this is not 2020."

www.ingramcontent.com/pod-product-compliance
Lightning Source LLC
Chambersburg PA
CBHW040521220526

45473CB00013B/2943